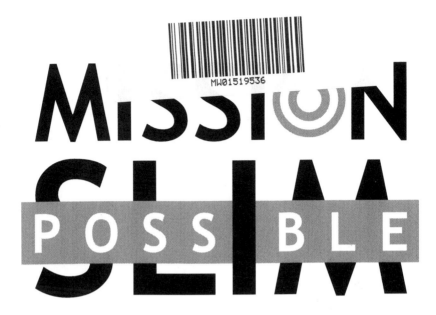

# MISSION SLIM POSSIBLE

## 10 WEEK DIET REVENGE

BY

ANDREA SEYDEL

*"Goals are just wishes without a mission (action) and a target (direction). Start Mission Slim Possible today"*

*- Andrea Seydel*

Published and Distributed in Canada by Life Balance Publishing Group, Inc.:
www.dietrevenge.com

Library of Congress Cataloging in Publication data

Seydel, Andrea

Mission Slim Possible: 10 Week Diet Revenge\ Andrea Seydel

1. Health, Fitness and Dieting-Non fiction 2. Self Help-Non fiction

Title ID: 4863928
ISBN-13: 978-1500248307

1st Printing August 2014. Printed in Canada

Cover Photo: Karolina Yen | kayphotography.ca

## PUBLISHER'S NOTE & DISCLAIMER

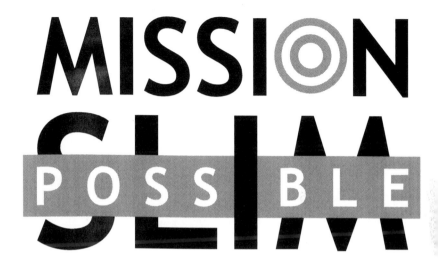

# MISSION SLIM POSSIBLE

## 10 WEEK DIET REVENGE

BY

ANDREA SEYDEL

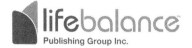

**lifebalance**
Publishing Group Inc.

# TABLE OF CONTENT

## WEEK ONE

*Awaken your inner power and live the life you desire.*
*Weight-loss starts in your mind.*

*Trim your waistline and improve your health by walking.*
*Walking is natural and good for you.*

*Are the common foods you eat causing you to gain weight? Make a switch*
*to natural, whole alternatives, and watch your waist slim down.*

## WEEK TWO

*Affirmations are powerful and the words you use can have impact*
*on your reality. Affirmations are powerful for living out your goals.*

*Surges or bursts of training can work wonders and gets results.*

*Alive foods, nutrient-dense foods, and cleanse days are important for*
*permanent weight balancing.*

# WEEK THREE

# WEEK FOUR

# WEEK FIVE

## WEEK SIX

## WEEK SEVEN

# WEEK EIGHT

*The psychological relationship you have with food plays*
*a huge roll on your Mission to slim. Banish cultural pressure,*
*deprivation thinking and gain psychological control.*

*Become a morning exerciser and be energized for the day.*
*Boost metabolism and fit your workouts in consistently.*

*The psychology of being slim and healthy and how it*
*relates to nutrition, food selection and control.*

# WEEK NINE

*Find happiness and acceptance of your self, while on*
*your Mission. Learn the benefits of managing your*
*expectations and stopping the tendency to compare.*

*Effective ways to lose belly fat with these tips and workouts*
*for a flatter stomach. Try some abdominal blasting challenges!*

*By keeping your blood sugar levels under control, you can*
*lose fat, regulate mood, and boost energy levels. Eating a lot*
*of fiber can help you to lose weight and regulate blood sugar levels.*

# WEEK TEN

*Self-hypnosis and using the power of your mind can help you*
*on your Mission. Program your mind for success!*

*Adopt a lifestyle of active living and recreation. Permanent*
*weight management is a lifestyle.*

*"If you choose to accept the Mission Slim Possible-you will be able to transform your life!"*

— *Maureen Hagan*

# FORWARD

# A REFRESHING AND INSPIRING APPROACH TO WEIGHT-LOSS

This book is a refreshing and inspiring new approach to one of the biggest challenges, and to date failures, the modern world faces - dieting to lose weight. This is not a diet book but rather a natural, holistic and practical approach to balancing your weight, maximizing your health and living a healthy and happy life. Being in the fitness and health care industry for 35 years I can honestly say that I have never read a book like "Mission Slim Possible" before. I was immediately captivated by Andrea's passionate and inspiring tone, extensive knowledge and the feelings of possibility that she projects through her writing. Andrea guides you through a 10 week journey one week at a time, and she breaks down the mission to become slim in a healthy way almost as if she was sitting right in front of you as your nutritionist, life coach and psychologist. This book equips you with tools and a step by step guide that will make you re-think your approach around food, dieting and life in general. It offers you practical solutions and skills that will effectively guide you through the process to attain a better and healthier lifestyle.

Andrea Seydel is the founder of Life Balance magazine and Publishing Group. Andrea has earned the reputation as being "an inspirational and optimal wellness coach". This book demonstrates and enhances that reputation. Her expertise and experience as a

Registered Nutritionist, Certified Life Coach and Fitness Professional, as well an author of a variety of self help books absolutely qualifies her to write this book. It's also evident by her lifestyle and positive outlook that she walks her talk and this will give you confidence that you are in good hands with Andrea as your coach. I know it is Andrea's mission in life to help as many people as possible to maximize their health and to live a balanced and happy life.

I am confident that if you care about your health and your life then you will buy this book, read it and if you follow its programs and adopt the attitudes set out in it you will achieve your goals! If you choose to accept the Mission Slim Possible- you will be able to transform your life!

In fitness and health,
Mo Hagan

Maureen Hagan - *Licensed Physiotherapist, Certified Fitness Instructor, VP Operations at GoodLife Fitness and Education Director for Canadian Fitness Professionals (canfitpro).*

*"Sometimes... the smallest drops in the bucket make the biggest ripples."*

*A.M. Hodgson*

# ACKNOWLEDGEMENTS: MISSION SLIM POSSIBLE

## To my fellow women,

I wrote this book for you, but when I began I didn't realize just how many women share in their struggle to feel good in their own bodies. You came to me craving realistic, authentic support and you said, "Why don't you make a book that packages up every thing you do and say?" I asked you what you wanted in that book, and you said, "loving support, guidance, and motivation to help me be myself again." You asked me to package my ability to make passion contagious, to give light to a sometimes negative subject matter and to inspire positive change. Well, here's your book. Nearly every tip, secret, and ounce of my encouragement is packaged into this book for you. You inspired and supported me and made this book a possibility for me. To the woman who so fearlessly, join me in my classes, attend my seminars, take my courses or have crossed my path, when we first met, my purpose began! I would like to express my gratitude to the many women who saw me through this book; to all those who provided support, talked with me, shared vulnerability and offered comments. You have given me the power to believe in my passion and pursue my dreams. I could never have done this without the faith you have in me. Thank you.

To my mother, Carole Seydel, I can barely find the words to express all the wisdom, love and support you've given me. I continually strive to be as good a mother to my kids as you are and always have been to me. Thank you for being my first introduction to healthy living, positive determination and recreation. It is all your teachings and role modelling that have moulded me and helped inspire my career. You're truly amazing.

To my special team of role models and friends who may or may not know the extent to which you have had a positive influence on my life; Maureen Hagan, Lara Miller, Alison Cur, Scotty Kearns, Stephen Rollick, Mike Leppard, Luis Alberto Pena Valdes, Judy Ornato, Sara Burton, Laura Gray, Simone Sheffrin, Leo Seydel, Alison Seydel, Jeff Seydel, Anthony Seydel, Wayne Dyer, Anthony Robbins, Peggy Cleland, Sherri McMillan, David Patchell-Evans, Liisi Tammor, Patricia Sica, Ina Brandts, Caroline Marie Dupont, Beryl Bender Birch, Desiree Sardo, and many many others. I beg forgiveness for all those who have been with me over the course of the years and whose names I have not mentioned. You too mean the world to me.

Last and not least: To my kids, Felicia and Damian, You bring me courage and happiness on a regular basis. You unconditionally accept, play and love me and for that I thank you. Your smiles, hugs and laughter are what I live for!

*"No one knows for certain how much impact they have on the lives of other people. Oftentimes, we have no clue."*

*Jay Asher*

# AUTHOR'S NOTE AND DISCLAIMER

Though the author and publisher have used their best efforts in preparing this book, they make no representations or warranties with respect to the accuracy or completeness of the contents of this book, and specifically disclaim any implied warranties or health claims or results for a particular purpose. At no time do the author or publisher suggest that the content of this book replace a primary care giver or replace medical attention and is not the substitute of a primary care giver for medical diagnosis or treatment or prescription of medication. The advice and strategies contained herein may not be suitable for your situation. You should consult with a professional where appropriate. Neither the editor nor the publisher shall be liable for any loss, damages, including but not limited to special, incidental, consequential, or other damages.

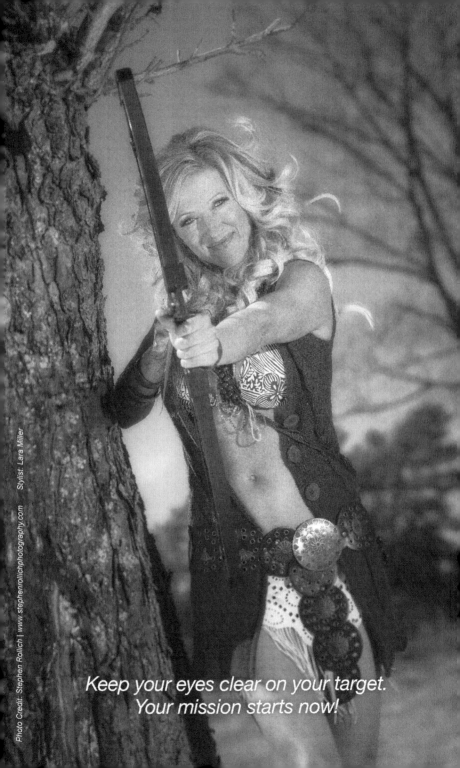

Keep your eyes clear on your target.
Your mission starts now!

# WELCOME TO MISSION SLIM POSSIBLE:

## Ten-Week Diet Revenge!

Finally the Mission that can help you get diet revenge once and for all! Being slim without dieting is possible and this program holds the natural path for you to take!

You did it! You have decided to stop dieting and take ownership of your health and well-being. Thank you for joining Mission Slim Possible: 10 Week Diet Revenge. This program is for diet liberation, personal effectiveness and transformation on all levels!

I invite you to be fearless and be the ideal you by taking the time to nurture your health. When you do, you will notice a genuine passion for life and a healthy awakening. You deserve to feel your best and in turn, everyone else around you will also benefit. You will quickly realize that this is a program like no other; it is a program based on losing and/or managing your weight the way nature intended. It is a program that looks at every aspect of positive health and weight management potential in order to achieve highly effective results. Mission Slim Possible is designed as a nutritional, psychological, recreational and lifestyle coaching program; putting results, focus and success at the forefront of the Mission. This program provides you with a week by week, unique approach to losing weight, by providing self-coaching and motivational tools to get your psychology in line with your target, tools to get you moving and exercising, and the knowledge to guide you on the right nutritional path, including the psychology behind weight management; as well as lifestyle adjustments and ways to inspire you and keep you motivated. You will lose weight on this program, but the focus, in addition to weight management, is to achieve a loving acceptance of your greatness and discover how you can improve your health and life balance overall. This program will equip you with the tools necessary to be successful on all levels. So, let us jump into a healthy life, filled with self-pride, passion, good choices, and self-care!

*You are in charge of your life and your Mission can create the positive changes you seek!*

Why is the majority of the population gaining weight? Why are people not getting results from magic diet pills, programs and exercise alone? It is because work and busy lives becomes a priority and a healthy diet and exercise drop off the list. Is it because quick fix magic pills are not enough and a more realistic approach needs to be taken for healthy results? As a society, we spend more time working, caring for others, wishing for easy options, and simply give up, or are in denial of the need for health management. Some people feel that their career is too urgent and there's not really time for self-care. But the truth is, without self-care we cannot sustain high quality work, take care of our families and loved ones, or feel proud of who we are. On top of all that, without self -care, we let ourselves go and we feel terrible as a result. Life is meant to be enjoyable and feeling great about your self is a big part of this happiness.

The good news is that you can alter your level of self-care. You can go on a Mission to get Diet Revenge and feel great doing it. You can use the knowledge presented in this book to achieve the success you dream of. It is, ultimately your decision to do everything in your power to change your reality. The choice is yours, the efforts are yours, and the determination is yours. You have already decided to follow a realistic, wonderfully holistic and natural approach by selecting this program. You've taken the first step on your Mission!

Mission Slim Possible: 10 Week Diet Revenge is, just that - a transformational Mission! My friends, family and clients often ask me, "Are you on a Mission or something?" The truth is, yes! I am often on a Mission of one kind or another to reach my goals and targets I set for myself. I am on a personal mission to educate, empower and help people through weight loss struggles. I have taken my life coaching, experience with clients, nutrition, psychology degree and fitness training to create this program for you. I have seen its success over the years and I know it can help you. It provides realistic and healthy solutions to all your weight management questions. It is transformational because it is effective and offers lasting results. It is a challenge because you need determination and desire to change your life for the better. This program is actually not a 'diet', but rather a collection of well-studied and successful approaches that will inform and educate you for a multi-faceted approach to weight balancing. Everything you adjust based on this program will combine and work synergistically to assist you on your path towards your Mission of being slim, healthy and sexy.

Follow this program week by week for ten weeks and focus on everything you can do during each week to achieve your goals. Each week builds on the week before. Be sure to complete each week accordingly, and with each section, I encourage you to track your success. I highly recommend keeping a journal. You will notice each week the program offers a life-coaching psychology section, recreation management section, and a nutrition section. Record your food intake, exercise regime (what you did and for how long), water consumption, and what motivated you. Remember, too, to write down your answers to the coaching questions from this program. Keeping up with your accomplishments is important; you put an amazing amount of effort into achieving greatness. Give yourself credit where ever and whenever you can!

Before you start, take a picture of yourself at your current weight. The 'before' photo will be used as a tool throughout the program. Seeing a truthful image of how you look prior to your mission and noticing the changes week by week is extremely motivating. I recommend wearing a bathing suit or fitness outfit for this photo. Stand in front of a full length mirror. Hold up your camera and snap a picture.

I invite you to jump into this program with both feet and enjoy the positive life transformation! You will feel wonderful reaching your goals every week and have a realistic outlook on nutrition, fitness and psychological wellness. By the end of the ten weeks you will be transformed on all levels. Stay true to your Mission and eyes clear on your target, track your progress and know whole-heartedly, slim is possible.

### Tips for success:

- Take your 'before picture'.
- Take Measurements, neck, waist and hips.
- Buy a journal or book to track your progress (there are a lot of cute options).
- This program is a collection of positive changes that work synergistically to ensure success. Be sure that you track everything that works for you as you go.
- Remember you are in charge of your life and you will create the positive changes you seek.
- Remember only you can make the changes you seek!

# WEEK ONE

## Psychology Management/Self-Coaching

Awaken your inner power and live the life you desire.
Weight-loss starts in your mind.

## Recreation Management

Trim your waistline and improve your health by walking.
Walking is natural and good for you.

## Nutrition Management

Are the common foods you eat causing you to gain
weight? Make a switch to natural, whole alternatives, and
watch your waist slim down.

*Mission Slim Possible: 10 Week Diet Revenge is a new natural holistic approach to balancing your weight.*

# — WEEK ONE —

## Psychology Management/Self Coaching:

Awaken your inner power and you can live the life you desire. Weight-loss starts in your mind

Welcome to week one of Mission Slim Possible. We need to reconsider the way we think about food and dieting. Rather than thinking about temporarily going on some hot new diet to shed weight or achieve some other aspect of wellness, we should be thinking about making achievable, realistic changes that we can sustain for a long period of time - like a lifetime!

So where do we stand? According to Statistics Canada, 67% of Canadian men and 54% of Canadian women are overweight or obese. These statistics are high, and they point to the ever-increasing problem of how to get people moving and eating healthy - and maintain a healthy and manageable weight. Often times, however, these statistics make headlines and the reaction can lead to finding a quick and often unhealthy way to lose weight. But, if you fall into this statistic, you need to remember that this is certainly not cause for shame. Everyone falls into unhealthy habits at some point in their lives. This is the purpose of Mission Slim Possible; to offer you solutions and skills to guide you through the process of better and healthier living. There is a way to naturally manage your weight and you are learning how on this program. This program is common sense, realistic and something you can do for life! The world has many pleasant things to offer and sometimes strength eludes us, but it's important to realize that a holistic approach to balancing your weight that is consistent and long serving is achievable. It should be mentioned that fitness and health go hand in hand, and that psychology or self-coaching are all important, and work synergistically, when balancing your weight. When a person is healthy, they are more energetic, more mentally acute, and often more confident! Your program starts here: and more specifically, starts with your mind!

Congratulations on joining Mission Slim Possible and getting diet revenge! You have decided to stop dieting and take ownership of your health and well-being naturally.

### Weight-loss Starts in your mind:

*"The greatest discovery of our generation is that you can transform your life by changing your mind." - Professor William James*

It may seem obvious that making daily healthy nutrition and fitness choices are a great way to manage your weight, and we will be addressing nutrition and fitness, but is weight-loss much deeper than that?

As a start to your mission every week, we have to get your mind prepared. You first have to decide you want to be slim, then really mentally desire to lose weight, as well as believe it is possible in order for you to reach your goals. We must use our minds and action in order to manifest and support the things we desire and dream. We must engage and take the right action to support and lead to the fruition of our goals, dreams, emotions and words. Only then can we awaken our inner power and positive attitude and live the life we aspire to! Your mission to be slim IS possible. Get diet revenge with these three mental tips to get you started.

## Connecting to your desire:

If you really want to be slim and desire this goal more than anything else in the world, you will hold the motivation to reach that goal. It is one thing to say "I wish I was slim", and it's another to really desire being slim and reach your goal. We all have goals and wishes and we all would love to achieve them. But what sets that person apart who seems to reach his goals and maintains priorities? It's a burning desire. How committed are you to achieving these goals? Under what conditions would you give up? What if you wanted to reach your goals so badly that you knew with certainty you would never give up? I challenge you to connect to your level of desire and when you are truly 100% committed to reaching your goals, you will move from hoping to knowing you can achieve them. You can either find a way or make one and do whatever it takes. To implement action, we must understand what we really want in order to bring happiness and success into our lives. Once it is clear to you what it is that you most desire out of life - the person you want to be - the success you want to enjoy - the health you need to thrive, then you are able to adopt the right strategies, make the right decisions and move toward achieving this life. Connecting to 'the why' you want to reach your goal can help you get a deeper burning desire to attain your goal. If you lack in the desire to be slim, even slightly, you will sabotage your attempts to reach that goal. A burning desire towards you goals will make a measurable difference in your life and help you establish clear, committed goals.

## Specify your target:

If you have realistic achievable expectations and specific realistic goals you will be successful. If you truly mentally desire weight-loss or a specific goal, nothing can stand in your way. Make sure you pick the right and realistic goal for you. This is an obvious point, sometimes we seem to put weight-loss at the top of our goal list but fail to factor in timing, specific expectations, and all the effort that is going to be required. Simply stating the goal isn't enough to be powerful. The only person responsible for your success is you. The first thing you must realize is that nobody else will do it for you. If you want to transform your life, you have to do it yourself - for yourself. Wow, right? This thought isn't meant to make you feel bad. On the contrary - it is meant to empower you. Take a moment to think about the goals you've set for yourself. Goals without a specific target, are like shooting a bow and arrows up in the sky, aimlessly. You must first decide exactly what you want to accomplish. Be as detailed as possible when setting goals. Give specific weights, dates, and times. Make sure you can measure your goals. For example; I lost two pounds in week one, two pounds week two, I increased my cardio to four times every week. I will be 20 pounds lighter by June 27. Goals must be in writing in the form of positive, personal affirmations of what you DO want and not what you don't desire. You can create the reality you want by deciding, first, what is it that you want your reality to look like. For example, if you desire a body like an athlete, start to think of yourself as an athlete, behave like an athlete, eat and train like an athlete, and before long, your dream will come true. Just like the athlete example, by acting like an athlete - exercising, eating right, staying determined, focused and positive, you will inevitably transform your body and mind into the athlete you desire to be.

The first step is to address the questions: "What do I want?" and "What reality do I see myself in?" The great part of this exercise is that you deserve to have exactly what you want in life and no one can stand in your way unless you let them. Change your attitude and focus on success and options. You can achieve what you really want simply by changing how you think and approach life. Whatever you decide to do today will make an impact or have an effect on tomorrow. Your efforts and good actions today are going to get you where you want to be tomorrow. Decide what you want and you will get it. Build into yourself the qualities needed to reach your goals. Create the reality you desire. Enjoy the process and try not to get wrapped up in the end results. It will come to you with love. Follow your dreams, goals and desires and you'll be amazed with how happy and successful you will be.

**Believe it is possible for you:**

*What ever your mind can believe you have the ability to achieve*

If you believe it is possible for you to reach that goal and see your success already you will be successful. Many of us are hard on ourselves and don't realize the attention we give the negative energy. Every time you look in the mirror and you say, "I look fat," or you say, "I'm not good enough," or "this will never work," you set yourself up to support that thought. This way of thinking inhibits our success with the program. This section is dedicated to help you transform those statements to look something more like these: "I am in the process of taking care of myself," or "I am getting slimmer and slimmer every day", and "I am proud of myself." Know that you can do it. If you asked most people how much they would love to complete and reach their goals, they would tell you how amazing that would be. Why do so many people fall short of their weight-loss goals, or any goal for that matter? Simple; they don't believe that they can, so effort and motivation fall short. You are the only one holding you back. As you look upon your life now, would you describe it as fun and exciting, or is it a lot of hard work? Would you describe yourself in great shape and healthy, or are you ashamed you let things get so out of balance? Do you tend to reach your goals easily, or do they seem to stay just out of reach, close enough to smell them, but never close enough to touch or achieve? Wouldn't it be nice if you could wave a magic wand and have the life and body you desire just like that? Well, it might not be that easy, but it can be a lot easier than you may think. Here is a wonderful part of the program that is very important to help you reach your goals and live the good life.

You can complete your goals. Yet until you firmly believe this, it won't happen. Take the time to visualize your goal and see yourself living your goal. this will make things more real and help you believe your goals can happen. Plan to do at least three things that support your goals every day. This will help you see progress and connect you to the belief it can happen for you. To succeed, we must first believe it is possible that we can reach our goals.

Consider these motivating statements by Rex Johnson and David Swindley from their book Awaken Your Inner Power:

- You create your own reality with your thoughts, feelings and attitudes.
- You have the right to a better quality of life: to health, happiness and success.
- The reason most people get ill is because their lives aren't working.
- You can transform your life by changing your attitude.
- Whatever your mind can conceive and believe, you can achieve.
- Decide to build into yourself the qualities and characteristics you need for success.
- You can have whatever you want in life, providing you are willing to invest the necessary time, energy and effort.
- Live in the present moment. Life is a journey to be enjoyed, not a struggle to be endured.
- Don't fight or rush life, everything will come your way when it is supposed to.
- Allow yourself to be guided and supported by the universal intelligence within and you will always be happy, healthy, successful and have the courage to follow your dreams.

*"In the long run, we shape our lives, and we shape ourselves. The process never ends until we die. And the choices we make are ultimately our own responsibility." - Eleanor Roosevelt*

We all have the ability to reach our weight-loss goals. Believe you can do it, set a specific plan, and connect to your burning desire to achieve them. Take immediate action once you set a goal for yourself and have worked through the desire, specifics and belief around your weight-loss goals.

### It's time for self-coaching and inner reflection:

Take time to answer and work through these questions in your journal to help keep you focused and on a clear path towards your goals. By taking action you will bring your goals into your life. These self-coaching questions will help clarify what you need to have accomplished this week.

### Self-Coaching Questions

- What needs to happen each day this week?
- What are my priorities this week?
- How will these action steps help me get closer to my goals?
- In the next week my complete focus will be on?
- My direction is clear to me because...?
- I am willing to commit to...?
- What might success look like to me for this week?
- What resonated and stood out to me from the program and what impact will it have on me this week?
- I deserve this because...?
- I am thrilled with myself because...?
- Why is it important for me to take action and follow my goals this week?

# — NOTES —

"*Walking is how the body measures itself against the earth.*"

— *Rebecca Solmit, Wanderlust: A History of Walking*

# — WEEK ONE —

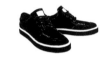

## Recreation Management:

Trim your waistline and improve your health with walking. Walking is natural and extremely good for you - it's nature's exercise program!

**Walk your weight off, It can be that simple:**

What low impact workout shapes and tones, energizes you, regulates your weight, is easy, fun and free? You guessed it...walking! For the first week on your mission, it is super easy to start increasing how much you move and walk. Whether you want to shed pounds or achieve a healthier you, walking is the easiest and most ideal exercise. Walking provides total aerobic fitness, efficient calorie burning, as well as strengthening and toning. It is amazing that something as natural as walking can have enormous health and fitness benefits! Start walking more this week and you will be addicted to walking and moving.

Walking is magical. After a few minutes of walking, you start to feel your shoulders relax, your chest open, your breath deepen, your legs awaken and your lungs feel full of fresh air. Best of all, you feel as though all your heaviness has been shaken off, and the day's activities fall away. Walking is a fantastic exercise for anyone - particularly those that suffer joint pain, have limited mobility, the elderly, pregnant women (I used walking everyday during and after both my pregnancies to help me bounce back into pre-baby shape), or someone with health issues that limit other forms of exercise, because it can be done without fatigue setting in. In fact, you feel more energized after a walk. Long duration, low intensity workouts, are particularly great for burning calories and fat without depleting too many of your energy stores. But weight loss is just one of the many health-related reasons to start a walking program. In fact, an American Heart Association study of 13,000 people conducted over 8 years, found that people who walked thirty minutes every day were at a much lower risk of premature death than those who didn't exercise regularly. Walking increases circulation (just ask my mom, who say shopping is good for her because it increases her circulation from all that walking, any excuse to shop!), it regulates your mood, heart-rate and blood pressure, it allows for your mind to open and therefore it can be a time for contemplation and reflection, and to de-stress.

While you don't have to walk fast to burn calories, your walk should be brisk to boost your heart rate and make it an aerobic activity. You want to challenge the heart muscle. However, if you are just starting a walking program, go easy, and slowly work up to a quicker pace. Of course, the longer, faster and harder you walk, the more calories you will burn and the more weight you will lose. But, remember, start slow and work at a pace that meets your health and fitness needs.

According to Health Canada the many benefits
of walking include:

- It is the most natural way to exercise.
- It is the very best way to start an exercise program. Even if you have never exercised, you'll be able to do it.
- It doesn't cost a cent.
- Your walk time is for you to enjoy. You can meditate, listen to music, and view your beautiful surroundings.
- You can walk alone or with friends and family.
- It is safe. It is almost impossible to get injured while walking.
- It is easy to adapt to your fitness level. Start out slow and build up gradually.
- Walking improves muscle tone, especially around the buttocks and hips.
- It promotes an overall sense of wellness. It is nice knowing you're doing something good for yourself.
- Walking is great for circulation and excreting toxins from your body.
- It is portable. You can do it anywhere - at home, at work or on holidays.
- It reduces blood cholesterol.
- It lowers blood pressure.
- It increases cardiovascular endurance.
- It enables the heart to pump blood to cells more effectively.
- It protects bones from osteoporosis.

- It increases bone density.
- It improves mood.
- It alleviates stress and depression.
- It stimulates endorphins (which helps you feel good).
- It increases energy levels and boosts metabolism.
- It assists in weight management.

The reason I included walking in the first week of Mission Slim Possible is because it is something you can implement right away and do through the entire program. This form of exercise does not require you to purchase expensive equipment or buy a membership. However, there are a few basics that you will need. It starts with shoes. Find a great pair of shoes that feel comfortable right away. Wear appropriate clothing. Select loose clothes that can be layered. The layer closest to your skin should be able to whisk moisture away from your body. A heart rate monitor, although not necessary for walking, can help you make your workout more effective. You can challenge your heart but not stress it either. A pedometer (or a step counter) is a fun, motivating gadget that can mark your progress.

Health Canada Suggests you remember safety when walking:
- Consider the weather and dress appropriately.
- Walk with a friend in areas that may be more secluded.
- Avoid wearing dark clothing at night.
- Wear reflective gear at night or early morning.
- Let people know where you are going and when you will be returning.
- Walk calmly past dogs or stop moving.
- Select walks where pathways are well lit and close to homes.

- When the weather is really bad, opt for a treadmill.
- When using an iPod or earplugs, keep the volume low enough that you can hear the traffic and people around you.

Living an active life doesn't have to mean going to the gym - every movement you make burns calories regardless of where and what you're moving. Park your car far away from an entrance, take the stairs instead of the elevator, stand instead of sit, make every effort to be in motion and move about. Although you need to take the opportunity to relax, try not to be lethargic. All movement burns calories, and all activities accumulate at the end of the day, resulting in weight balance and/or maintenance. Walking just happens to be an easy, effective, natural way to balance weight and improve your health.

### Try this ten-week walking program:

This ten-week walking program will help you burn calories, improve circulation and help you get fit and healthy. Studies recommend that you exercise a minimum of five days a week for thirty minutes a day. Walking is a great way to accomplish this requirement. This program guides you to your goals, including longer walks and speed work. Feel free to accommodate the walking program to meet your needs and how you feel. Walk at a brisk pace and you should be slightly out of breath, but still able to talk. Walking with a friend or listening to music are great ways to pass the time and motivate yourself.

*Remember: Keep a log or record in your journal your walking to track your progress week to week and maintain your momentum.*

# Weeks One & Two:

Walk for 15-25 minutes four to five days per week.

# Weeks Three & Four:

Walk for 30 minutes three days per week and 40 minutes once per week.

# Weeks Five & Six:

Walk for 30 minutes three days per week and 60 minutes once per week.

# Weeks Seven & Eight:

Walk for 30-40 minutes three days per week and 60 minutes once per week.

# Weeks Nine & Ten:

Walk for 45 minutes at a moderate pace, two days per week and 60 minutes slow once per week. Plus, do a 30-minute speed walk once per week: Warm up for five minutes, then alternate three minutes fast, three minutes slow for 20 minutes. Cool down five minutes. Spend some time figuring out when it is best for you to walk and build it into your weekly schedule.

The invention of the automobile, although hugely convenient, has made walking a bit of an archaic form of transportation. I am not suggesting that you throw away your car keys, but I am recommending that make a point of building walking into your daily or weekly life. After all, it's what your body is built to do. I promise you that if you follow the program, you will see how your actions will pay off in a very positive way. For one, you will notice a huge difference in how you feel and how your pants fit when you start walking more. Perhaps you're thinking that walking for a set period of time is too difficult at first. Perhaps then, you fit in short, unscheduled walks in when and where you can. Maybe it's while your daughter is in gymnastics, or it's during your lunch break; maybe it's while you're waiting for someone at an appointment, or, as my mother suggests, it's while you're shopping! You get the picture! Walk whenever and where ever you can. The accumulation of your little walks count, and they add up to your overall fitness level. My personal favorite time to walk is after my kids go to bed, I hop on the treadmill and get caught up on my emails. Walking is always good for you, no matter how often or how you do it. Just try your best, get out and walk…and remember to have fun! Move it and you will lose it. Walk the pounds away and stay healthy.

*"Adopting a new healthier lifestyle can in-volve changing diet to include more fresh fruit and vegetables as well as increasing levels of exercise."*

— Linford Christie

# — WEEK ONE —

## Nutrition Management

Are the common foods you eat causing you to gain weight? Make a switch to natural, whole alternatives, and watch your waist slim down.

### The secrets behind nutrient debt foods:

In this day and age, processing and refining is the common practice with our food industry. There are so many foods that are not found in the state that nature intended. Rather, it has become the norm to find foods that are over-processed and lacking in nutritional value and fiber. These are sometimes referred to as fraction foods, because they contain a fraction of the original product. Examples include (but are not limited to) non-whole grain wheat, packaged or canned foods, and foods that contain refined sugars. We are busy people, with demanding lives. We see more and more households juggling a work-life balance poorly, particularly when both parents (or partners) are in the workforce. It is a challenge, to say the least, to find the time to cook and prepare foods from scratch that are healthy and whole. The result is an over-consumption of fraction foods that are ready-made for convenience. The trouble with these foods is that preservatives and additives have to be added and much of the goodness and life force taken out.

What you have to remember is that the food processing industry isn't necessarily concerned with our health and well-being. Conversely, manufacturing of food is driven by profits. How can they produce a mass quantity of food that tastes good and keeps consumers coming back for more? According to Food Matters and Hungry for Change, the food manufacturers remove the parts of foods that slow down production (such as the germ part of a grain) and that increase spoilage, and add a whole bunch of additives and preservatives. Most fiber is eliminated, as are the vitamins and minerals, because all these are what normally cause the foods to spoil quicker, and instead, preservatives are added to keep the product on the shelf much longer than nature intended. Let's keep going. Packaged food is more often than not made with an unhealthy load of salt and/or sugar to make the product more desirable and tasty. And, just to make sure it tastes good and looks good, they add chemically derived additives to boot. In the end, these processed, packaged foods are full of all of the wrong ingredients and none of the right ones!

Fraction foods are processed foods, lacking in any real nutritional value.

When you eat foods that are deficient or void of vitamins and minerals, the body has to make up and, provide for the absence of nutrients, resulting in your body experiencing a nutrient debt. Nutrient debt leads to weight gain and poor health. The body is very smart and seeks a state of homeostasis, which is a state of equilibrium, and it will create cravings for more food. In other words, when you are nutritionally starved, your body naturally seeks more food resulting in excess calories. And, if the foods you consume are not the right foods, you are then consuming far too many more nutritionally void calories, resulting in unhealthy weight gain. So, you become not only calorically starved, but nutritionally starved as well. And, what happens to all of these excess calories? They are stored in your body as fat if we do not use up the excess amount of calories.

When nutritionally starved, your body naturally seeks more food resulting in excess calories.

The removal of vitamins and minerals in our foods is one problem. The other is the removal of a very vital part of many whole foods - Fiber! Fiber is essential to ensure proper bowel function, to create a feeling of fullness, and to regulate your blood sugar. When fiber intake is limited, you end up with a sluggish functioning bowel and this leads to bloating and toxic overload. Moreover, fiber is vital in controlling your blood sugar levels. It slows the absorption of sugar into the blood. The absence of fiber in your diet causes blood sugar levels to rise too quickly and the result is an excess of insulin being secreted. Insulin's role is to take sugar out of the blood and put it into your cells. This insulin overload results in a sharp drop-off in your blood sugar. When your blood sugar levels are too low, you may feel anxious, depressed, hungry, or stressed. Your body will respond to these feelings by putting glucose (blood sugar) back into your blood from stored glycogen in your liver. You essentially experience a yo-yo effect with blood sugar levels that leave you with excess fat storage and ups and downs in energy. When our cells are full and no more glucose is needed, the glucose combines with the insulin and is stored as fat. In summary, the lack of fiber in food destroys the body's ability to properly regulate sugar. You end up storing fat, having mood fluctuations, and eating more - all of which contributes to further eating, a stress response and ultimately weight gain.

Remember, food that enters your body with no nutritional value will steal vitamins and minerals from your body, leaving you nutritionally starved and needing more food. These fraction foods are lacking in essential fiber to keep your blood sugar levels in check and your bowel system working properly. If you continue the cycle of adding more fraction foods to your body, the result is an excess of calories and fat storage and ultimately weight gain. All food that has been processed and refined creates a nutrient debt and calorie excess.

According to the Academy of Nutrition and Dietetics, the over-processing and refining of foods is the reason the majority of the population is gaining weight and having health issues, such as diabetes.

**The power of nutrient dense foods to manage your weight:**

The most important strategy to develop while on your path to healthy living is to decrease the nutrient debt and replenish your body with nutrient dense foods. By choosing foods that are in as close to their natural state as possible, you will ensure that you are getting all the goodness that Mother Nature intended. By eliminating processed foods, you will be eliminating those foods that create that nutrient debt. Remember, you end up overeating, craving food, and using up your precious nutrients already in your body! Alternatively, when you eat nutrient dense foods all the calories that you consume are full of nutrients and lead you to good health and proper weight management. When foods come into your body with full nutritional value and fiber, your body instinctively knows how to deal with this food. Your digestive system works optimally to allow for a gradual rise in blood sugar and a gradual fall. The body uses up the calories and nutrients appropriately, providing your cells and organs what they need to function properly, and as well, you crave food appropriately.

Natural nutrient dense foods are the secret to shedding weight and keeping your weight and health managed well.

**Get diet revenge on sugar:**

It may or may not come as a surprise, but one of the most highly processed and refined foods, which lack nutritional value and natural fiber, is sugar. Sugar is highly consumed and appears in many food products. Manufacturers refine sugar to make it available to many industries and prevent it from spoiling. Refined sugar is very stable and like most purified chemicals will keep indefinitely. The modern industrial processing of sugar consists of two stages: First, they crush sugar cane at the mill and press it many times to create granular sugar.... Secondly, the juice is chemically treated to remove some impurities, bleached and then boiled down (losing many nutrients) until it begins to crystallize, leaving sugar. Refined white sugar is hidden in a lot of our everyday foods such as cereal, breads, condiments, and sauces. According to the FDA Statistics show that the average person eats double their weight in refined sugar each year. Refined sugars have neither nutritional value nor natural fiber and is therefore, simply, empty calories. When you eat refined sugars, you incur a debt and therefore have to consume the corresponding quantity of vitamins, minerals, fat, protein, and fiber to make up for the nutrient debt. Brown sugar is white sugar with molasses poured on top and while this returns a tiny amount of nutritional value to the sugar, it still is not a healthy sugar choice.

It's not easy to cut out sugar unless you have alternatives and the good news is that there are many other natural sweeteners to choose from that have full nutritional value. Genuine natural raw sugar is made by evaporating the water from sugar cane juice and allowing it to solidify and granulate. Raw sugar cane is the best form of sugar. Natural sweeteners are foods that are natural, and provide complete nutritional value and natural fiber. Natural sweeteners can replace refined white sugar. Using natural sweeteners as an alternative to white sugar will provide you with nutrient dense, fiber rich natural options.

---

### Natural Sweeteners options:

| | |
|---|---|
| Honey | Nut butters |
| Pure maple syrup | Unsweetened applesauce |
| Raw sugar cane | Demerara |
| Sucanat | Raw sugar cane |
| Agave | Natural jam |

---

The list of sweeteners provided in the list above are also low on the glycemic index, which means they have a gentle effect on your blood sugar levels. Natural sweeteners keep your blood sugar levels consistent, your energy and emotions stable, and help you sleep properly; all of these are essential for positive weight management. By eating natural sweeteners your weight, mood, and energy will be properly regulated.

## Wheat verses whole grains, what to get revenge on:

Wheat products are mass produced and mass consumed. Grains, such as wheat, are spoiled if they are not in their natural state. Grains are supposed to be eaten whole. There are three parts to a grain of wheat: the germ, the endosperm and the bran. The germ houses all the nutritional value such as vitamins and minerals. This part of the grain upon germination and sprouting gives rise to tiny leaves and rootlets and contains the life force and the nutrients of the plant. The endosperm or the bulk of the grain contains the protein and much of the gluten content that makes breads springy. The bran or tough outer coating protects the grain and is indigestible by humans; because it is indigestible it acts as a good fiber. When processed, the germ and the bran are extracted leaving the endosperm. What you're left with is flour that has little or no fiber, vitamins or minerals; a flour source that no longer is natural. Due to the fact that no nutrients are being provided in refined wheat, your body has to make up for what is not available to it, resulting in the stealing of nutrients from your system for digestion and utilization. Just like with sugar, your body has a nutrient debt and does not feel satisfied. In a recent experiment done at McGill University by Professor Joe Schwarcz, Director of the McGill University office of Science and Society, rats fed a diet of only commercial enriched white bread showed stunted growth and two thirds of them died of malnutrition within 90 days. Because of the refined nature of the wheat, the food no longer has healthy, beneficial fiber to move properly through the body creating a sticky, clogging tendency instead. There is a faster rate of absorption into the blood due to lack of nutrients and fiber – this in turn upsets your blood sugar levels, your mood and causes cravings for more refined sugar or wheat. If you satisfy your cravings with the same type of food, the end result will be excess calories and weight gain. Since the flour is no longer the way nature intended it to be, it has dangerous effects on the body.

You may be asking if whole-wheat flour counts as a refined flour? It does. In Canada, when wheat is milled, parts of the kernel are separated and then recombined to make whole wheat flour. Under the Food and Drug Regulations, up to 5% of the kernel can be removed to help reduce rancidity and prolong the shelf life of whole wheat flour. The portion of the kernel that is removed for this purpose contains much of the germ and some of the bran. However, according to the American Association for Cereal Chemists International definition, it is only when all parts of the kernel are used in the same relative proportions as they exist in the original kernel, that the flour can be considered whole grain. In Canada, according to Health Canada, it is legal to advertise any food product as "whole-wheat" with up to 70% of the germ removed. While the resulting product will contain the benefit of fiber in the nutritional information, it lacks the nutritional content found in the wheat germ.

Whole grains contain all three parts of the kernel - the germ, endosperm and bran. Examples include rolled oats and brown rice. Canadian consumers can be assured of whole-grain products by a label stating 100% whole-grain whole wheat. Eating grains in their natural state - the state that nature intended - has a profound effect on health and weight management. Whole grains are full of nutritional value and enter your body with full fiber and nutrients. Avoiding wheat can be a tough endeavor unless you know what to use as a replacement. There are many whole grain options to keep the nutritional value and fiber levels where they should be.

## Healthy whole grain options:

Oats                    Brown rice

Rye                     Kasha

Bulgur                  Millet

Ancient grains *(such as spelt, quinoa, amaranth, teff, and Kamut)*

## Some alternatives to wheat:

There are some direct health benefits, along with weight management advantages, to switching to alternatives to wheat. Almond flour, for example, is higher in protein, fiber and vitamin E. It's also higher in nutrient-dense carbohydrates, so it's excellent for managing weight and blood-sugar levels. Almond flour is raw, blanched whole almonds that have been ground into a fine powder, so it's a great substitute for any baked goods. Spelt is getting a lot of publicity these days, and for a good reason. Considered an ancient grain (meaning, it's a grain that has been unchanged for millennia), it's very high in protein, a form easier to digest than the form found in wheat, as well as higher in fiber and B complex vitamins. Similarly, quinoa flour is jam-packed with nutrients. According to Experience Magazine, quinoa is known as the "gold of the Incas", and offers twice the amount of protein as most cereal grains, and is an excellent source of fiber, calcium, iron, magnesium, phosphorus and riboflavin.

Many of the above-mentioned grains come in pastas, breads, cereals, crackers, and flours. Eating these foods will fill you with the nutrients that you need to feel satisfied and function properly throughout your day. These foods provide great consistent energy from its full fiber source; it will keep your bowels and blood sugar levels regular. When food enters the body with natural fiber and nutrients, it enters the body and blood at a steady rate. Studies consistently show that when natural fiber is ingested at a higher rate from natural foods, the body weight tends to be lower than a diet low in natural fiber. The more natural fiber you consume, the less weight you gain and the more weight you lose.

Natural, nutrient dense foods are the secret to shedding weight and keeping your weight and health managed. It's worth repeating: by choosing foods that are as close to their natural state as possible, you will ensure that you are getting all the goodness that Mother Nature intended.

Keeping track of what you are eating is also very important with this program. Be sure to fill out a weekly food chart in order to monitor what you are eating. There are fantastic apps for your phone that can help you with this. This process will make you aware of what you consume and make you accountable for your results. Search for a great app which appeals to you to record what you eat or simply keep a food journal or record of what you eat.

### Sample options shopping list: For natural sweeteners and whole grains:

Here is a sample list for shopping that uses whole grains and natural sweeteners. These are just suggestions. Visit your health food sections in your grocery store or go to a health food store where you can find all these wonderful natural sweeteners and whole grain products. There are so many varieties, brands and options now available at health food stores and grocery stores that are not listed here. This is an introduction to the wonderful world of whole foods.

| SUGGESTED ITEMS | BRAND IDEAS | SUGGESTED ITEMS | BRAND IDEAS |
|---|---|---|---|
| Raisons | PC® Organics™ food line | Mayonaise Nayonaise | Na Soya Caroline Nutrimax |
| Apple Sauce | PC® Organics™ food line | Flax Seed Oil | Omega Nutrition |
| Raw Honey | Brosia® | Pumpkin Seed Oil | Omega Nutrition |
| Nut Butters Apple Butter | Almond Budder Mara Natha Nuts to You | Hemp Seed Oil | Manitoba Harvest |
| Brown Rice Syrup | Lundberg® | Balsamic Vinegar | Bionaturae |
| Maple Syrup | | Veganaise | Earth Island |
| Jam | Crofter's Organic Natur le Fruit | Salt & Herbs | A.Vogal Simply Organic |
| Herbal Teas | Yogi Tazo | Buttery Spread | Verve Earth Balance |
| Miso Soup | Kome | Soy Sauce | Bragg's |
| Nori Dried Seaweed | Koyo | Tamari | San J |
| Soups | Imagine Amy's | Seeds & Nuts | Omega Nutrition Sunridge Farms |

| SUGGESTED ITEMS | BRAND IDEAS | SUGGESTED ITEMS | BRAND IDEAS |
|---|---|---|---|
| Rice | Lundberg® Casbah | Nut Bars | Natura Life |
| Beans | | Fruit Leathers | Kettle Valley |
| Quinoa | Eden | Molasses | Wholesome |
| Apple Cider Vinegar | Omega Nutrition | Cane Sugar Sucanat | Wholesome Sweeteners |
| Salad Dressings | Ruth's Organic Ville Simply Natural | Yogurt | Liberte Organic Meadows |
| Cereals- Kamut Corn, Spelt, Millet, Rice | Nature's Path Sunny Crunch Nature Path | Bread- Rye, Rice, Spelt | Stonemill Dimpflmeier Kinnikinnick |
| Hot Cereal & Oats | Bob's Red Mill Nature Path Earth's Best | Pasta- Kamut, Rice, Spelt | Artesian Acres Udon Rizopia |
| Granola | Bear Naked | Flour- Rice, Barley | Oak Manor Bob's Red Mill |
| Milk | Organic Meadows | Apple Butter | |
| Rice, Soy, Almond Milks | So Nice Silk, Ryza, Natura | Drinks- Pure Juice | R.W Knudsen Kiju, Just Juice |
| Tofu | Nutri Bio Sol Cuisine | Smoothies | Arthurs Fresh Com. |

We all have the ability to reach our weight-loss goals. Believe you can do it, set a specific plan, and connect to your burning desire to achieve them. Take immediate action once you set a goal for yourself and have worked through the desire, specifics and belief around your weight-loss goals. Trim your waistline and improve your health with walking. Walking is natural and extremely good for you - it's nature's exercise program! Make a switch to food choices that are natural, whole alternatives, and watch your waist slim down. As a start to your mission this week, you have to get your mind prepared. You first have to decide you want to be slim, then really mentally desire to lose weight, as well as believe it is possible in order for you to reach your goals. It's going to be a great week for you. This is just the start!

# STAY ON TARGET

| MY WEEKLY CHECKLIST | MY WEIGHT THIS WEEK: |
|---|---|

## MY WEEKLY CHECKLIST

- ☑ Walk Daily
- ☑ Choose Natural Sweeteners
- ☑ Choose Whole Grain Alternatives
- ☑ List Desires
- ☐ _____
- ☐ _____
- ☐ _____
- ☐ _____
- ☐ _____
- ☐ _____
- ☐ _____
- ☐ _____
- ☐ _____
- ☐ _____
- ☐ _____
- ☐ _____
- ☐ _____
- ☐ _____

## MY WEIGHT THIS WEEK:

Began at:_____

Finished at:_____

Total weight loss:_____

## MY MEASUREMENTS THIS WEEK:

### BEGAN AT

Shoulders:_____

Chest:_____

Waist:_____

Hips:_____

### FINISHED AT

Shoulders:_____

Chest:_____

Waist:_____

Hips:_____

### DIFFERENCE/TOTAL INCHES LOST:

Shoulders:_____

Chest:_____

Waist:_____

Hips:_____

What really resonated for me this week?

_____

_____

_____

_____

_____

_____

_____

_____

_____

What worked well for me this week?

_____

_____

_____

_____

_____

_____

_____

_____

_____

_____

# WEEK TWO

## Psychology Management/Self-Coaching

Affirmations are powerful and the words you use can have impact on your reality. Affirmations are powerful for living out your goals.

## Recreation Management

Surges or bursts of training can work wonders and gets results.

## Nutrition Management

Alive foods, nutrient-dense foods, and cleanse days are important for permanent weight balancing.

"The most important words are the ones we utter to ourselves, about ourselves, when we're by ourselves."

— *Anonymous*

# — WEEK TWO —

## Psychology Management/Self Coaching:

Affirmations are powerful and the words you use can have impact on your reality. Affirmations are powerful for living out your goals.

Welcome to week two of Mission Slim Possible! This week will allow you to explore how you can use affirmations to drive positive change, both in your weight-balancing approach as well as in your life overall! Since affirmations and words can enrich and change your life for the better, it is fitting we address this early in the program. Affirmations are positive, specific statements that help you to overcome self-sabotaging and negative thoughts. This mental skill will have a strong impact on your weight, recreation and life management level of motivation. Remember in week one we talked about desire? If you really want to be slim and desire this goal more than anything else in the world, you will hold the motivation to reach that goal. Affirmations and the power of your words will take this level of desire to the next level.

## The power of affirmations:

*Do you ever say to yourself any of the following type of statements?*

- "I'm never going to be able to be slim; I'm just not athletic enough."
- "Why does my boss want me to present at the trade show? I'm a terrible public speaker, and I'll just embarrass the company."
- "I wish I could look after myself, instead, I let others walk over my time and needs."
- "I'm never going to reach my goals."

Many of us have negative thoughts similar to these, sometimes on a regular basis. When we have these thoughts, our confidence, mood and outlook become negative as well. The problem with these negative thoughts or statements we tell ourselves, is that they can be self-fulfilling. We talk ourselves into believing what we think is true and the outcome is that we feel inadequate. And, because of this, these thoughts drag down our personal lives, our goals, and our careers. Our very thoughts can sabotage our efforts and desired goals. This is why consciously doing the opposite - using positive affirmations - can be helpful.

This section of Mission Slim Possible will allow you to explore how you can use affirmations to drive positive change, both in your weight-balancing approach as well as in your life overall!

## Why use affirmations?

Affirmations are positive, specific statements that help you to overcome self-sabotaging and negative thoughts. They help you visualize, and believe in what you're affirming to yourself, helping you to make positive changes to your life. You can use the power of affirmations to create everything you desire for yourself. Tell yourself you are becoming slim and healthy and you will achieve this.

Affirmations are statements you give yourself that programs your subconscious mind and assists it in becoming a reality in the conscious waking state.

Crazy, you might say? When I was taking psychology at university it was explained to me in this way: when you were learning how to drive a car, you had to consciously focus on what needed to be done. You learned by being conscious or aware of what to do. After a while, it became easy to the point where you didn't even think about putting the car in gear. You get to the point where your subconscious mind drives the car for you. Learning new things has to start in the conscious state. By programming or feeding in the affirmations in the waking state, you are thus programming a new reality for your subconscious mind - a state that you desired and made from your affirmations. Affirmations are conscious, deliberate requests made in the conscious state. The options are limitless. You can develop strength and a new reality for yourself from the power of affirmations. You literally decide what you want to program into your mind.

*"You become what you think about most of the time."*
*- Brian Tracy*

Telling yourself the same positive message over and over again can harness previously untapped power in your mind. Over time, the repeated affirmations recognized by your conscious mind begin to penetrate your subconscious. It then creates images of new experiences, and manifests your new desired results. You coach yourself towards your goals, programming your subconscious mind to create the new desired results. When you say mean-spirited or negative things to yourself, you damage your self-confidence and limit your potential for success. You create a negative experience for yourself. Every time you catch yourself saying something negative about yourself, start counteracting it with two positives or even delete it in your mind.

## The science behind affirmations:

Wondering if affirmations really work? While there's limited research into the effectiveness of using affirmations in a general setting, there is evidence that the use of positive affirmations can successfully treat people with low self-esteem, depression, and other mental health conditions. As well, it has been proven effective in goal setting and acquisition. For instance, in a study by researchers at Northwestern State University, people who used positive affirmations for two weeks experienced higher self-esteem than at the beginning of the study. Also, two different studies, one published in the Journal of American College Health and one conducted at the University of Kentucky, Lexington, found that women treated with cognitive behavioral techniques, which included use of positive affirmations, experienced a decrease in depressive symptoms and negative thinking.

Current trends in neuroscience offer evidence that we can consciously improve our health and well-being by simply changing our thoughts. "Discoveries in 20th century neuroplasticity have demonstrated that the physical reality of our brain has been formed from our past experiences and can change based on new input", says Danea Horn author of the book 'Chronic Resilience'. Lauren Robins, (MS, LMT) in the article, 'The Indefinite Body' says, "Thoughts create chemicals that pour into the rivers and streams coursing through our body. Within 20 seconds, the chemical composition of the body is altered by a thought, having an acid or alkaline effect on our body... As we persevere on limiting negative thoughts, our nervous system sends chemicals to muscles; our physical body contracts and thinking becomes foggy." Deb Shapiro, the bestselling author of 'Our Body Speaks Your Mind' says that there is now a whole new science called "psychoneuroimmunology", which explores the relationship between the psyche or mind, the nervous system and the immune system. In this book, she poses an interesting question: "Do you ever wonder how the power of your thoughts can affect your body?" She gives the example of Dr. Bernie Siegel, the author of 'Love, Medicine and Miracles', who was giving a talk to a room full of skeptical doctors when he brought out a copy of Lady Chatterly's, 'Lover', and proceeded to read the most erotic portion of the book. As he put the book down he said, "Just as reading a book can stir our sexuality, so you can see how our thoughts and feelings can affect us physically." The doctors were immediately convinced!

Some people may view affirmations as "wishful thinking," or simply looking at the world with an unrealistic perspective. Quite a lot can depend on your mindset. The bottom line is that thought is power and affirmation thought is energy and can affect us on many levels. Try looking at positive affirmations this way - many of us do repetitive exercises to improve our body's physical health and condition. Affirmations are like exercises for our mind and outlook; these positive mental repetitions can reprogram our thinking patterns so that, over time, we begin to think and act in a new way. Not for anything else, affirmations make us feel good and better about our self and life.

**When to use positive affirmations:**

You can use affirmations in any situation where you'd like to see a positive change take place. These might include times when you want to:

- Raise your confidence before presentations or important meetings.
- Control negative feelings such as frustration, anger, or impatience.
- Improve your self-esteem and confidence.
- Finish projects you've started.
- Stay focused on the goals you set.
- Improve your productivity.

Affirmations are often more effective when they're paired with other positive thinking techniques and goal-setting techniques (we will discuss this more in weeks to come. Affirmations have been proven useful when setting personal goals such as natural weight balancing. Once you've identified the goals you'd like to achieve in the short and long term, you can use positive affirmations to help keep yourself motivated in order to achieve them.

**How to use affirmations:**

Remember - affirmations are positive statements that help you challenge and overcome negative thinking and self-sabotaging behaviours. They are usually short, positive statements that target a specific area, behaviour, or belief that you're struggling with. Start by thinking of the areas of your life you'd like to change. For instance, do you wish you had more willpower? Perhaps you want more meaningful relationships with your friends? Do you want a more productive day? Write down several areas or behaviors you'd like to work on. Then, for each of these, come up with a positive, present-tense statement you can repeat to yourself several times a day.

It's also important that your affirmation is credible, believable, and based on a realistic assessment of facts. For instance, imagine you feel bad about the rate of pay you're currently receiving. Then you begin to use affirmations to raise your confidence about asking for an increase. However, it probably wouldn't be wise or realistic to affirm to yourself that you're going to double your salary: for most people, and most organizations, doubling what you're earning just isn't feasible. Try to keep it realistic!

Repeat positive affirmations to yourself three times in the morning and three times at night. Say the affirmation out loud with emotion. Look in the mirror and look deep into your own eyes as you affirm. Write down your affirmations and repeat them over and over again during the day. Use flash cards. Record yourself saying your affirmations and listen to them. Before you know it, your subconscious mind will be programmed the way you desire it to be. You can find all kinds of affirmation applications for your phone as well. My personal favourite applications and books relating to affirmations are by Louise L. Hay by Hay House and Oceanhouse Media. Many of the following affirmations have been influenced by Louise L. Hay, one of my mentors around the area of affirmation and positive thinking.

Examples of positive affirmations

I have plenty of ideas to reach my goals!

My efforts will be recognized in a positive way by my friends and family!

I can do this!

My opinion is respected and valued by others!

I am successful!

I am determined in my life, and my work!

I like putting effort in and reaching my goals!

I'm grateful for the health I have!

I enjoy focusing on my wellness!

I'm bringing a positive attitude to myself every day!

I am excellent at what I do!

I am generous and caring!

I am happy!

I will exercise strong self-control!

**Positive thinking affirmation:** Today is a great day. I look great. I feel successful. I attract success and notice all the good around me.

**Health affirmation:** My health gets better and better each day. I feel strong and healthy. My body heals itself. I am a completely healthy person.

**Energy affirmation:** I feel energized. Power is flowing through me. I have passion and enthusiasm for life. My energy and enthusiasm brings me complete success!

**Positive body image and confidence affirmation:** I have a strong healthy body. I look fantastic. I look after my body. I take time to nurture myself. I feed myself healthy foods. I am at a perfect weight. I look slim and healthy. I have great confidence. I am proud of my body. I love myself!

### Now create your own:

The advantages of making your own affirmations are that you can personalize them and make them specific to you. These are easy for the mind to absorb which makes them quite effective. Create at least three and put them on cue cards to read daily. Remember, if the affirmations are not realistic, your subconscious mind will reject them. A good way to start your affirmation is by stating: "I am in the process of ..." The use of affirmations is just one way to make positive changes to your life.

When making your own, remember:

- Affirmations are positive statements that can help you overcome self-sabotaging and negative thoughts.
- To use affirmations, first analyze the thoughts or behaviors you'd like to change in your own life and career.
- Next, come up with positive, credible, present tense statements that are the opposite of your negative thoughts.
- Repeat your affirmations several times a day, especially when you find yourself slipping into a negative thinking pattern, or engaging in a negative behavior.
- Remember that affirmations are most effective when used alongside other strategies, such as visualization and goal setting.

### It's time for self-coaching and inner reflection:

Take time to answer and work through these questions in your journal to help keep you focused and on a clear path towards your goals. By taking action you will bring your goals into your life. These self-coaching questions will help clarify what you need to have accomplished this week.

### Self-Coaching Questions

- What needs to happen each day this week?
- What are my priorities this week?
- How will these action steps help me get closer to my goals?
- In the next week my complete focus will be on?
- My direction is clear to me because...?
- I am willing to commit to...?
- What might success look like to me for this week?
- What resonated and stood out to me from the program and what impact will it have on me this week?
- I deserve this because...?
- I am thrilled with myself because…?
- Why is it important for me to take action and follow my goals this week?

# — NOTES —

*"Lack of activity destroys the good condition of every human being, while movement and methodical physical exercise save it and preserve it."*

— *Plato*

# — WEEK TWO —

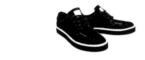

## Recreation Management

Surge and burst training can works wonders
and gets results.

Are you tired of your monotonous cardio routine? Not achieving the fitness results you once were? Fitness classes feel intimidating and long? Or do you simply put off working out entirely due to lack of time? If you answered yes to any of the questions, then surge or burst training could be just what you need. Burst training is basically high intensity interval training and has been gaining popularity basically because it has great benefits.

## What is surge training?

Dr. Josh Axe, author of Burstfit: The fastest way to get fit, explains burst training as one of the fastest ways to get lean and toned. He says short surge or burst interval training has long been a part of an athlete's regimen. And now fitness professionals and trainers say that it's gaining popularity with the general population because it gets results fast. Since shaking up workout routines is essential, and spending time at the gym isn't always possible, short bursts or surge intervals of fitness can get you amazing results to naturally balance your weight. Burst training is high intensity, short duration exercise that causes the body to respond with increased hormone production and a physiological response needed to burn fat and produce muscle even after you've completed your workout. It's minimum time with maximum results. Surge training is designed to push the body to its maximum ability for a short period of time as opposed to longer, slower paced workouts, such as running or walking on a treadmill. Contrary to popular belief, more is not necessarily better. Surge training is a great tool to naturally balance your weight particularly when you find it a challenge to find time to exercise. Best of all, when using surge training, the body feels energized and will continue to burn fat and build muscle hours after the short activity.

## How does surge training help you on your Mission?

Several studies have confirmed that exercising in shorter bursts with rest periods in between burns more fat than exercising continuously at a moderate rate for an entire session (despite the fact that longer, endurance style workouts result in a higher caloric loss overall). Endurance training may provide the calorie burn you are aiming for, but burst training will create the right hormonal responses for real fat loss and lean muscle development. According to Keighlagh T. Donovan, group ex-athlete trainer, high-intensity intervals, such as those used in burst training, has been proven to stimulate growth hormones and testosterone, both of which are powerful fat burning hormones. Another benefit to burst training is that it does not over-stress the body as sometimes seen with overtraining or exercising excessively. Long duration exercise, such as hour-long workouts at the gym is not natural for the human body. The human body burns fat for energy or "fuel" and as a result, it will make and store more fat for the next endurance workout. Our bodies are very smart with long duration workouts and will store more fat in case that long duration workout happens again. Please note this does not apply to lower intensity workouts such as walking, which is very natural and effective. Burst training, on the other hand, teaches your body to recover quickly and build lean muscle tissue in preparation for its next intense workout.

Burst training is particularly appealing to those who are significantly overweight or are not very fit, since the short spurts of interval-based movements encourages the idea that you do not have to work very long before recovery or rest is granted. Of course before you start anything new, you must consult with your physician. Although burst training requires that you must push yourself to your maximum potential during the short intensity period, it psychologically seems more bearable than the thought of attempting to run consistently for sixty minutes. The reason it is great for Mission Slim Possible is that it is attainable, doable, and realistic to stick with while balancing your weight. The other fantastic advantage of this style of workout is that no gym or equipment is needed. Simply running stairs, doing push-ups, or doing "air" squats for twenty to forty-five seconds (three to six reps) is all you need to do.

### How do you do surge/burst training?

At this point you may be wondering what exactly a burst training style workout would actually look like. Assuming you are aware of proper form and technique, you may easily draw-up a quick program based on your capabilities and background knowledge of exercise. If you are unsure of your abilities or form, it is always recommended that you first speak with your doctor or health professional and research some exercises before attempting anything new or unfamiliar. Choose any large rhythmic motion such as a run, jog, jump, jack, dance, hill climb, etc., and alternate effort phase with recovery phase and do this for fifteen to twenty minutes in total.

Surge training examples:

- Run in place for 35 seconds as hard as you can
- Rest For 90 seconds
- Run in place for 35 seconds as hard as you can
- Rest for 90 seconds
- Run in place for 35 seconds as hard as you can
- Do 10 reps of 35 seconds run, 90 seconds rest, for a total of 20 minutes (Vary the exercise (e.g. run) so you don't get bored)

*Congratulations- you will now burn fat for the next 24 hours!*

### 20- minute surge/burst ideas for workouts

Always start with a light warm up. Choose an idea from the list below and perform each set of five exercises with as little or no break between exercises for 20 minutes, three times per week. You can start to create your own and mix a bunch of moves.

## Idea#1

- Mountain climber (as long as you can or for 35 seconds)
- Pushups (as many as you can)
- Squats jumps (10-12 reps)
- Bicycle crunches (as long as you can)
- Box Jumps (or you can run in place) 30 seconds
  Rest (90-120 seconds) REPEAT for 20 minutes.

## Idea#2

- Jump lunges (as many as you can)
- Dumbbell reverse flies (10-12 reps with each arm)
- Forward lunges (12-15 reps with each leg)
- Dumbbell squat and presses (10-12 reps)
- Jumping jacks (or run in place) 30 seconds
  Rest (90-120 seconds) REPEAT for 20 minutes.

## Idea#3

- Close grip pushups (as many as you can)
- Triceps dips (as many as you can)
- One legged bends (10-12 reps with each leg)
- Two arm dumbbell raise (15 reps)
- Wide squat jumps (or run in place) 30 sec

Rest (90-120 seconds) REPEAT for 20 minutes.

**Surge training steps to get you going on your Mission:**

- Make a commitment to yourself that you are going to make exercise an important part of your day. All you need is 20-30 minutes three days a week to see dramatic health benefits.
- Begin to perform Burst/Surge Interval training style of exercises.
- Plan the workouts into your schedule.
- Remember even 10 minutes of Surge training will be better than no training.

*You got this...*

*"The better you eat in terms of quality,
the better you will feel as a whole. "*

— *Andrea Seydel*

# — WEEK TWO —

## Nutrition Management

Alive foods, nutrient-dense foods and cleanse days are important for permanent weight management.

Our approach to week two nutrition management will involve an understanding of which foods are the best choice to maximize your health and improve your ability to shed pounds and maintain a healthy weight. In this section, I will introduce you to alive foods and how cleansing is a key component to weight management and detoxification.

### The power of foods that are Alive:

When you consume alive foods you can't help but feel full of life. Alive foods are foods that have not been overcooked or processed and still contain all the natural vitamins, minerals and enzymes needed for vitality. They are great for counteracting a nutrient debt by providing many nutrients with lower calories. Moreover, they are essential to assist in weight loss and natural weight balancing. We are suffering from an over-processed and unprecedented chemically contaminated diet; it is refreshing to think that we might totally reverse the whole picture by recapturing a natural, uncooked or raw, alive foods diet - eating the way nature intended! Fruit and vegetables are alive foods and therefore an excellent choice to include in your diet. These foods have the sun's energy, minerals from the soil and energy from the universe. Nuts and seeds that remain in their natural state are considered to be alive as well. As you eat alive foods, the energy and vitality from these foods transforms to become energy and strength for you.

How you cook (or not cook) your vegetables is very important! By heating food, the starch in the cell membrane swells and ruptures, allowing precious vitamins and minerals to leak out or become destroyed. Once a cell's membrane is damaged, it is subject to oxidation damage from the air. For this reason, food should not be kept for long periods of time before being eaten. Vegetables are best eaten raw or lightly steamed or sautéed - avoid overcooked, canned, older leftover food. Raw, alive foods help improve digestion and bloating because they contain many enzymes and natural fiber. Enzymes are essential for good digestion and every bodily process. Raw foods are wonderful for a weight loss regimen because the fiber content makes you feel full along with regulating bowel activity and toxin removal. Moreover, raw, alive foods provide a low-calorie, highly nutritious addition to your diet; a definite bonus for natural weight balancing and health promotion! Alive foods flood the body with vitamins and life force. You are left with ample energy, balanced emotions, and weight loss or weight balancing. Alive foods give rise to healthy cells and healthy cells keep your constitution strong. A healthy constitution wards off illness and keeps you balanced. When you keep your food choices alive, you are sure to get all the vital nutrients needed to be healthy and maintain a balanced weight. When blood sugar levels are gradual you have consistent energy and store less excess blood sugar as fat.

*TIP: Each day, try to ensure your diet is made up of 75% alive foods. This means fruit all morning, nuts and seeds in your yogurt, a large salad with lunch, snacks of raw vegetables, and at dinner, eat an array of steamed vegetables. It is easy to do and will saturate your body with nutrients, fiber and enzymes - all of which are essential to maintaining your weight naturally and keep you healthy.*

Good quality foods will change the quality of your life. The better you eat in terms of quality, the better you will feel overall. If you treat yourselves like a sacred temple, your bodies will love you in return. The best thing the community can do for their health and the environment is to select foods grown organically. This is the way Mother Nature intended you to eat.

*The better you eat in terms of quality, the better you will feel as a whole.*

### Adding a lighter 'cleanse' day to your week will help you get diet revenge:

When on Mission Slim Possible, it is important to counteract the damage done in the past that caused the weight to creep on. A day of cleansing to saturate your body with nutrition is a good tool to improve health on all levels and manage weight naturally. One of the secrets to natural weight balancing is to balance your nutrient deficits created in your body. Since it is a deficit of nutrients and an excess of calories that contributed to weight gain in the first place; it makes perfect sense to expose the system to an abundance of nutrients and fewer calories to lose the excess weight.

If you want to lose weight you need to flood your system more regularly with nutrient dense foods and avoid any days with excessive calories and foods that cause nutrient debt. You can do this by giving your body just one cleanse day per week of nutrient-dense, low-calories. To counteract the nutrient debt, you need to look at these days as a fantastic method of keeping your weight balancing effective. Remember, it is not a starvation day, but a nutrient saturation day. You do not want to put the body into conservation mode and slow your metabolism. You need to ensure that you are eating large quantities of the suggested foods all day long. Consider this a cleanse day filled with alive foods that are nutrient-dense and full of natural fiber. Pick one day in your week when you know you will be successful. You will continue this cleanse day weekly for the rest of the program. This can be done in the future as well for general maintenance and good health.

### On cleanse day eat:

- Fruit & Vegetables
- Brown rice, in moderation (if you need some substance)
- Drink large amounts of water with lemon
- Diluted fruit juices (that do not contain any added sugars or chemicals)
- Smoothies (without yogurt)
    You will notice how this cleanse day will set the stage for healthy

eating and fill your system with ample vitamins and minerals to function well. These nutrients come in with few calories and facilitate weight loss and/or management. Be sure not to go more than two hours without eating. Try to stick to fruit in the morning and vegetables all day long. Enjoy the feeling of saturating your body with life force and nutrients. This day is like pressing the reset button.

## What to expect on this cleanse day:

When you cleanse your body there are many other benefits beyond nutrient saturation. When we consume foods that enter the body with life force and nutritional value, we give the liver and body a break from digestion. Did you know that digestion takes more than 80% of your body's energy? If you remove the pressure of digestion from your body, you allow the liver to do all its other jobs, such as mobilizing fat out of the body more effectively. When your body's energy is not focused on digestion, we have more energy to burn calories. This can be achieved by eating alive foods. Think about it this way; when you wake up in the morning there are tell-tale signs that your body has spent the night cleaning up shop. The corner of your eyes has accumulated rheum (sleep), you have 'morning breath', and you have to urinate. When the body is not in digestion mode, it can do these other jobs such as assimilate nutrients where needed and eliminate waste – this is a process that happens during the night when you are not eating. This can happen during the day as well when we consume alive foods that give your body a break from having to break down hard to digest foods. Instead, it can purify and cleanse your body effectively. In addition, the large amount of fiber that comes in with fruit and vegetables benefits your bowels, regulates your blood sugar levels and moves fat (such as cholesterol) out of your body.

Studies show there is a correlation with an increase in natural fiber (fruit/vegetables/nuts and seeds) with a direct decrease in weight. When the body can put energy into assimilating, eliminating and cleaning the blood, every part of the body will benefit. Your physical body has the natural ability to heal itself. When we remove the obstacles to good health, your body can do its natural thing; sustaining your life with quality. Your body will not waste energy on digestion; instead you will have more energy to burn calories and lose weight.

You can cleanse even if you are at your desired weight. Think of it as a weekly tune-up for your body. Enjoy cleansing one day a week while you are on the program, and it will likely become a nice habit you will not want to stop.

This week will allow you to explore how you can use affirmations to drive positive change, both in your weight-balancing approach as well as in your life overall! Also, surge or burst training is a great tool to naturally balance your weight particularly when you find it a challenge to find time to exercise. Adding a day of cleansing to saturate your body with nutrition is a good tool to improve health on all levels and manage weight naturally. Remember, when you consume alive foods you can't help but feel full of life.

Take this time to connect with your goals you'd like to achieve in the short and long term, you can use your positive affirmations and word selection to help keep yourself motivated in order to achieve them. Best of luck and stay determined and on track!

# STAY ON TARGET

## MY WEEKLY CHECKLIST

- ☑ Plan time for surge training
- ☑ Add a cleanse day
- ☑ Eat more alive food
- ☑ Make short term goals
- ☑ Say and use affirmations
- ☐ _____
- ☐ _____
- ☐ _____
- ☐ _____
- ☐ _____
- ☐ _____
- ☐ _____
- ☐ _____
- ☐ _____
- ☐ _____
- ☐ _____
- ☐ _____
- ☐ _____

## MY WEIGHT THIS WEEK:

Began at:_____

Finished at:_____

Total weight loss:_____

## MY MEASUREMENTS THIS WEEK:

### BEGAN AT

Shoulders:_____

Chest:_____

Waist:_____

Hips:_____

### FINISHED AT

Shoulders:_____

Chest:_____

Waist:_____

Hips:_____

### DIFFERENCE/TOTAL INCHES LOST:

Shoulders:_____

Chest:_____

Waist:_____

Hips:_____

What really resonated for me this week?

_____
_____
_____
_____
_____
_____
_____
_____
_____

What worked well for me this week?

_____
_____
_____
_____
_____
_____
_____
_____
_____
_____
_____

# WEEK THREE

# Psychology Management/Self-Coaching

Visualizing, is realizing your potential. If you can see and feel your success you can reach your goals.

# Recreation Management

Group exercise can give you that extra push and motivation to reach your weight balancing goals and keep you on your Mission.

# Nutrition Management

It's not just what you eat but how you eat that affects where your weight wants to balance. Discover how eating properly and controlling portions can lead to diet liberation.

*"Visualizing is daydreaming
with a purpose."*

— *Bo Bennett*

# — WEEK THREE —

## Psychology Management/Self Coaching:

Visualizing is realizing your potential. If you can see and feel your success, you can reach your goals.

Welcome to week three of Mission Slim Possible! This week will allow you to explore how you can use visualization to drive positive change, both in your weight-balancing approach as well as in your life overall! By creating a picture of your goals in your mind and keeping that image fixed, you have the capability to turn that image into a reality. The only person responsible for your success is you. The first thing you must realize is you need some idea or image in your mind of what specifically you desire for yourself. If you want to transform your life, you have to do it yourself - for yourself. Creative visualization is a technique to harness the power of your mind to create something you desire. By creating a picture of your goals in your mind and keeping that image, you have a good chance of staying motivated, on your Mission and connected specifically to what you desire for yourself; capable of turning that image into a reality. In week one we talked about goals without a specific target being like shooting a bow and arrows up in the sky, aimlessly. You must first decide exactly what you want to accomplish. Be as detailed as possible when setting goals. Visualization takes this idea of specifying your goals to the next level.

**Visualizing is realizing getting you closer to your target:**

What you see is what you get. You are moving forward, exploring new pathways to success. The effort you make each day is a direct investment in your future for health and well-being. The power of visualization is an effective tool that is as easy as daydreaming. By creating a picture of your goals in your mind and keeping that image fixed, you have the capability to turn that image into a reality. Once the recognition and visualization process happens, the image of that goal on your mental screen begins to link new thoughts and ideas in your brain, all related to a single goal.

**What is visualization and how can it help with your Mission?**

Creative visualization refers to the practice of seeking to affect the outer world by changing one's thoughts and expectations about the reality. It is a basic technique underlying positive thinking and is frequently used to help individuals attain the goals they seek. Visualization is a creative technique of using your imagination to visualize specific behaviours and events that you desire to have manifest into your life. Advocates suggest creating detailed visualizations of what you desire and see it in the mind's eye over and over again with all your senses. For example, in sports a gymnast may visualize a perfect routine over and over again to mentally train muscle memory. One of my favourite uses of visualization is for giving flawless speeches. I don't write my presentations, I simply visualize what and how I am going to present over and over in my mind until it is the way I want the speech to be delivered. Then on speech day, it comes out exactly the way that I envisioned it. Intense focus will help make your goal a reality. You are what you think about most of the time. If you say you are fat; you will be. You begin to believe it, you eat like you are, and you behave like you are. The opposite is also true. Convince yourself that you are an athlete, and you will eat like one and train like one. Visualization is the extension of the power of thought. Putting pictures on your mental screen and then concentrating on them takes the natural process a step further. The more visual and the more emotion you attach to the image, the more effective your visualization will become.

### Some science behind visualization:

In one of the most well known studies on creative visualization in relation to sports, according to Integral Health Services, Russian scientists compared four groups of Olympic athletes in terms of their physical and mental training ratios. Group one received 100% physical training, group two received 75% physical training with 25% mental training, and group three received 50% physical training with 50% mental training. Group three had the best performance results, indicating that certain types of mental training, such as visualization, can have significant measurable effects on performance. Studies continue to support that mental images can act as a prelude to behaviours. It is now widely understood and accepted in neuroscience and psychology that subjective training can have a direct involvement in consciously desired outcomes. One of my favourite books about creative visualizations is by Shakti Gawain (2002) "Creative Visualization: Use the Power of Your Imagination to Create What You Want in Your Life." This book provides powerful tools to help you use visualization to create the life you want.

*"You must see your goals clearly and specifically before you can set out for them. Hold them in your mind until they become second nature." - Les Brown*

Your imagination is your greatest gift. Imagine a life without limits. Creative visualization is a technique to harness the power of your mind to create something you desire. If you desire to be fit, healthy, slim and sexy, you can use visualization to make your dreams come true. You use visualization every day, though you are probably not totally aware that you use it. When you daydream, or conjure up pictures of food, friends, or anything you think of, you are using visualization. Visualization is a powerful tool to naturally manage your weight. It harnesses the power of your mind - body connection. Before you can lose weight or reach any other goal for yourself, you must be able to see yourself doing it in your mind's eye. Visualization can focus your mind, catalyze your emotions, and provide powerful motivation to keep you on track towards your weight balancing goals. Visualization can help you manage cravings, portion control and food selection when you are managing your weight. Researchers have found that the brain cannot actually tell the difference between something imagined and something real. As talked about in Week One of the program,

Visualization is a great tool to use to evoke the power of the Law of Attraction. By visualizing yourself as a slimmer, healthier, stronger person, your subconscious will begin to believe you are this person. Your subconscious will begin to assist you in achieving your goals. You will then begin to act according to your visions. As you begin to focus on your positive intentions around weight balancing, you will begin to attract experiences and behaviours that are aligned with your intentions. As a result, you will feel more motivated to balance your weight, choose healthy nutrient dense foods, and exercise more. Experiences and people will show up in your world to assist you in achieving your goals. You will find yourself more interested in healthy foods. Your outer reality will begin to conform or align with your inner reality.

**Projects to help you start and use creative visualization:**

1. Journal snapshot of visualization - Take time everyday to visualize your goals clearly - notice as much as you can about this picture you are creating. What are your desires? What are your behaviours? What are you wearing? Where are you? What makes you feel successful? What do you see? What do you feel? What do you hear? What do you smell? How do you define your success? Once you have your vision of success, take a snap shot of it and write up a detailed description of this in your journal. This image is always changing so don't stress over it being perfect. Read and visualize this image daily to keep you moving towards the successful achievement of your goals!

2. Your Mission vision board - Once you have a clear vision of yourself at your ideal weight, you will want to make a vision board of the new self you want to create. This is the time to let your imagination

go crazy. Let yourself dream up a new self and new life for yourself. A vision board is a collage and visual manifestation of something you want to bring into your life. It is a potent reminder and tool that creates a strong visual of what you desire. It sets the stage and your intention for creating a new life for yourself. Use the power of your imagination to create the life you really want. Cut out pictures from magazines or copy from Google Images that depict the life you want for yourself. Paste these images on a board or piece of paper. Cut out pictures of clothes styles, hairstyles, and accessories you will wear at your ideal weight. Cut out pictures of people near your ideal weight - pictures of people enjoying the lifestyle you want for yourself, the activities that you would like to do once you reach your ideal weight. These pictures can represent the work you would like to do, vacations you'd like to take, etc. Don't hold back. Let yourself go and notice the feelings associated with every picture you choose. Envision the life you desire for yourself.

### Points to help you remember:

- The mind is extremely powerful.
- It can be used as a tool to transform your reality by convincing your subconscious how great you will be.
- Use affirmations to reach your weight balancing goals.
- Creating a personal visualization is powerful.
- Visualizing creates the image you want and implants it strongly into your mind.
- This is a powerful tool to reach your specific outcome.

*You can do it...*

**It's time for self-coaching and inner reflection:**

Take time to answer and work through these questions in your journal to help keep you focused and on a clear path towards your goals. By taking action you will bring your goals into your life. These self-coaching questions will help clarify what you need to have accomplished this week.

## Self-Coaching Questions

- What needs to happen each day this week?
- What are my priorities this week?
- How will these action steps help me get closer to my goals?
- In the next week my complete focus will be on?
- My direction is clear to me because...?
- I am willing to commit to...?
- What might success look like to me for this week?
- What resonated and stood out to me from the program and what impact will it have on me this week?
- I deserve this because...?
- I am thrilled with myself because…?
- Why is it important for me to take action and follow my goals this week?

# — NOTES —

*"It is health that is real wealth and not pieces of gold and silver."*

— Maureen Hagan, VP Operations, GoodLife™ Fitness Clubs

# — WEEK THREE —

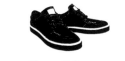

## Recreation Management

Group exercise can give you that extra push and motivation to reach your weight balancing goals and keep you on your Mission.

**Group exercise classes are powerful for motivation:**

As kids, we loved to play with our friends and get together with others. As teenagers, our world revolved around friends and social events. As adults, we still enjoy being active with friends, but don't always have the time or opportunities. Group exercise can provide that opportunity to feel young, have fun, and be physically fit with others. Group exercise is typically described as exercise performed as a group, with individuals led by a qualified instructor.

A variety of group classes exist, including (but not limited to) aerobics and dance choreographed to music, Pilates or core conditioning, yoga, muscle conditioning, step, spinning, kickboxing, boot camp and Zumba. Your choice of class depends on the club or studio you attend, the instructor's delivery, and the amount of time you have for your workouts. According to the American College of Sports Medicine and Lorna Sloukji from canfitpro (Canadian Fitness Professionals), group exercise offers a variety of benefits you might miss out on if you choose to work out on your own.

If you need that extra push to join a group exercise class. GoodLife Fitness Canada, gives ample number of reasons (below) why you should start participating in action-packed classes filled with warm smiles, great tunes, and an inspirational instructor!

**1. Strengthen your heart and lungs** - Cardiovascular exercise delivers oxygen and nutrients to your tissues, helping the overall circulation of blood through your heart and blood vessels. When your heart and lungs are working better, you'll find that you can approach your day with more energy and enthusiasm.

**2. Get better sleep** - We've all experienced that seemingly endless night trying to fall asleep. By amplifying your physical activity during the day, you'll be able to fall asleep faster, wake up refreshed and face the day with improved concentration and an enhanced mood.

**3. Manage your weight** - If you want to shed some extra pounds for the summer season, you have to get off that couch and move your body! By working out in a group environment with others who most likely share similar fitness goals, you'll be more inclined to keep up with your regime, helping you accomplish your weight goals.

**4. Improve your sex life** - Regular exercise leaves you feeling and looking better, giving you more confidence and a willingness to open up to your partner. And, with better circulation, you can achieve more satisfying sex.

**5. Make friends** - The gym is a wonderful, social place buzzing with energetic people. By consistently heading to your group exercise classes, you'll notice other regulars, start chatting before or after class, and foster good friendships. Make it a ritual to go out with a few people from your group exercise class every week or two, and keep each other motivated to reach your goals!

**6. Keeps you motivated and interested** - A common reason given for quitting an exercise program is boredom. A variety of class formats will keep you motivated and interested, as well as give you different instructor styles, music selection, and interaction with other participants. For many, an hour-long workout goes by very quickly when there is music playing and you are trying new exercises. People stay interested because of the social atmosphere provided by group exercise. This offers camaraderie and accountability among participants, as well as between participants and instructor.

**7. Appropriate for all levels** - Group exercise classes offer workouts from beginner to advanced levels. Participants do not need to know how to develop a safe and effective workout or which machines to use or for how long; it is already done for you. You simply have to show up with a positive attitude, participate, and most importantly, have fun!

**8. Structure and purpose** - An exercise class structured with a purpose can be beneficial to those with limited knowledge about safe and effective exercise programming. An appropriately designed class includes warm-up, cool-down and flexibility, in addition to the conditioning section. When you exercise on your own, you often skip portions of a workout you know less about or are not a favorite to perform. Furthermore, the fitness professional is not only designing the components of the workout, but also the intensity, so the class is designed appropriately to improve cardiovascular and muscular fitness. The fitness professional can also serve as a resource for class participants and encourage you to engage in other healthy behaviors outside of class.

**9. Consistency in schedule** - Consistency in scheduling offered by group exercise programs allows you to choose the class and a time that best suits your daily life and to stick with it each week. And, with all of the friends you've made in the class, you are motivated to attend to stay accountable and to keep up with them socially!

**10. Diversity to meet your interests** - Group exercise appeals to many people because of its diversity. Traditionally, group exercise was available inside a fitness facility in the format of dance choreographed to music. While this still exists, many non-traditional group exercise formats are emerging, some even outside. There are boot camps at your local park, yoga on the beach, ski conditioning at the soccer field, trekking on the bike trails, stroller-walking classes in your neighborhood, and Latin dance at the local recreation facility. Regardless of your passion or interest, what is most important is to move. Group exercise offers an outlet for people to do this while having fun!

Since group training has proven to be super effective with motivation and managing weight, it seems like a great choice to naturally balance your weight. There are many options now to meet your interests, time constraints, and fitness level. Your challenge for this week is to find some drop-in classes, or if you belong to a gym already, join the group ex-craze! Classes keep things fun and uplifting as well as benefit us socially, mentally, physically and emotionally.

*"Take care of your body. It's the only place you have to live."*
*- Jim Rohn*

"If we eat too little, we know it. If we eat too much, we know it. But there is a calorie range, or "mindless margin", where we feel fine and are unaware of small differences... over the course of a year, this mindless margin would either cause us to lose 10 pounds, or to gain 10 pounds."

— Brian Wansink

# — WEEK THREE —

## Nutrition Management

It's not just what you eat but how you eat that
determines where your weight wants to balance.
Discover how eating properly and controlling
portions can lead to diet liberation.

**Mindless eating & digestion: Why we eat more than we think:**

Do you catch yourself eating fast and mindlessly? Do you sometimes forget or fail to realize what you have put into your mouth? With
busy schedules, distractions and convenience foods, this is not uncommon. The way you eat could be giving you extra calories and therefore,
the pounds can slowly creep on. By slowing down and eating mindfully,
you not only improve digestion you will eat less calories.

When you eat quickly and mindlessly, your digestion is hindered and you don't realize what or how much you have consumed. When you eat your food, your body literally surrounds it. Though the food is in the digestive tract, it is still not 'in the body'. While some nutrients penetrate the intestinal lining and enter the blood stream, others may travel the length of the digestive tract without being absorbed. Two people eating the same diet may end up with dramatically different intakes of protein, fat, carbohydrates or other nutrients. When you eat quickly and mindlessly you are less likely to properly digest your food. This lack of digestion ultimately leads to excessive eating and weight gain. In addition, the food tends to ferment and putrefy, resulting in food for micro-organisms in the large intestine, which manifests itself as bloating, gas and/or constipation. We need and want nutrients to enter the body so we can feel satisfied and benefit from the health of the good nutrients that enter our system. How we eat relates directly to weight management and our health, but we must first understand the process of digestion to really understand the impact.

**The process of digestion and it's impact on your Mission:**

Chewing your food is where physical digestion starts. It is important to chew your food thoroughly, breaking it down into small manageable sizes for the body. Digestion actually starts in the mind's eye. Just thinking of the food you will eat will prepare the body for what is coming soon. Your salivation starts and enzymes are secreted. I'll never forget the time my brother had an infection in his salivary gland, strange, I know, but he said to me holding his cheek, "stop talking about food, your making my mouth hurt." It shows that just thinking of food stimulates the digestion process and since his glands were infected he could feel them when they were doing their job!

Chewing your food into a paste before it enters the next stage of digestion will allow the brain to prepare the body for the food entering into your system. When we slow the eating process down, the body has the chance to prepare for digestion and allow for a sense of being full or content (and therefore you eat less). The sense of taste also plays a big role. Taste along with sight and smell seems to "program" the digestive process for a sequence event of enzymes, proteins and acids secretions as well as the mental realization of eating food. Since digestion actually starts in the mind's eye, thinking of food and imagining it within the mind becomes a very important part of digestion. By maintaining a slow and steady intake of food, your body can digest food better and allow nutrients to enter your blood stream and subsequently your cells.

*Taking your time and realizing what you are eating will cause you to eat less, absorb more nutrients and feel satisfied.*

The liver plays a big role in digestion. Simply put, the liver is your biochemical mastermind. It is the metabolic director of incoming food and waste. It filters all blood, nourishes cells, stores and regulates sugars, processes protein, makes bile to absorb and digest fat, eliminates fat, and takes toxins out of your body. Those are just a few of the plethora of jobs the liver performs! In terms of weight loss, the liver is very important as it metabolizes fat in and out of the body; it regulates energy levels as a result of blood sugar levels, takes toxins out of the blood and allows the bowel to work efficiently. The liver works best when digestion is good. It is important to chew your food slowly and thoroughly, eat in a calm and relaxed environment and avoid overeating so as not to bog down the liver. When food is not digested well, the liver has to do a lot more work, and jobs such as energy regulation, fat metabolism and detoxification, are sacrificed. These are the jobs that are key to weight management! When your liver has to work all night digesting and assimilating food, it has little or no time to cleanse and detoxify, leaving the body sluggish and tired. Being sluggish and tired is not a good thing for burning calories and balancing weight.

**Slow down and eat mindfully:**

Slow down and eat mindfully and you'll eat fewer calories, improve digestion and appreciate what is going into your body. Proper digestion and mindful, slow eating has a great impact on weight management. It takes your body twenty to thirty minutes to realize that you are eating or have eaten. If you eat quickly and mindlessly, you can see how it is easy to overeat. If you finish eating quickly, you will still feel hungry because your brain has not had the opportunity to tell you that you are full. This feeling of satiety, or distention of the stomach, or feeling of satisfaction with what you have eaten, takes time to communicate this message to your brain. Eating slowly will allow the liver to absorb B vitamins, which are essential to proper metabolism, energy production and fat mobility out of the body. When we eat mindfully and slowly our systems work optimally, and we are therefore able to deal with anxiety and stress and prevent overeating and weight gain. OH MY GOODNESS! Can you see the huge impact of 'how' you eat on your health and weight balancing?

It is highly recommended that you make a conscious effort to slow down and enjoy your food with all your senses. Remember, 80% of your energy is needed to digest your food. When you are stressed, you are not in digestion mode. Instead you're in stress response mode, and being in this mode while you eat will prohibit proper digestion, and in turn poor nutrient absorption, ultimately leading to poor overall health. I have dedicated Week six to stress effective eating. For now, avoid eating while under stress. Try to relax and eat in a calm, relaxed state of mind.

*Numerous studies have shown that if you slow down your eating, you will consume on average 50% fewer calories!*

The bottom line: When you slow down your eating, you will improve your digestion, improve absorption, increase health and added nutrients, eat 50% fewer calories, feel more satisfied, experience little bloating or gas after meals, have more energy and feel great! Now that's fantastic!

### Tips to slow down and eat mindfully

- Eat in a calm and relaxed environment. If you eat when the television is on, or have commotion around you, your ability to focus on eating will be diminished and you will not be aware of what and how much you are consuming.
- Avoid eating when you are emotionally upset. When you are upset, you are in a different state of mind, one that is not conducive to eating and digesting.
- Avoid eating in stressful situations. When you are in stress mode your body is not putting energy into digestion, but rather into dealing with the stressful circumstance.
- Avoid drinking large quantities of liquid with your meals. When you over-consume liquid, you dilute the acids and enzymes. These are produced to help you digest your food.

- Try proper food combinations. The theory is that protein takes anywhere from four to 12 hours to digest. Starch takes anywhere from three to six hours to digest. If you eat these foods together you will add the digestion time together and ultimately you lose a lot of energy in digestion mode. You also fatigue the body in this regard and something will be sacrificed. Food will not break down effectively, leading to fermentation and putrefaction. Avoid eating protein and starch together. Instead, eat proteins with vegetables, starch with vegetables, and eat fruit alone.

**Additional ideas to consider applying to your Mission:**

- Fast for 14-hours a day. This will give your body a break from digestion and allow for cleanup and weight-loss (most of this time you are sleeping).
- Connect to your food with all your senses and a greatful attitude.
- Realize the gift you receive from the universe every time you eat. Slow down and appreciate your food.
- After eating one helping, wait twenty minutes before having a second helping.
- Slow down and you will eat 50% fewer calories.
- The fewer calories you eat the more weight you will lose.
- When you slow down your eating, your body can digest food properly.
- It takes your body twenty to thirty minutes to realize you have eaten.
- Eating slowly allows us to be aware of what and how much we consume.
- Poor digestion leads to poor liver function and therefore poor fat metabolism.

- Eating slowly allows us to feel satisfied with less food.
- Slow down and watch your weight fall off!

### Portion control is diet liberation:

Since when did extra large become so extra large? Our super-size servings are becoming so increasingly large it is hard to know how much we're really eating! I call my new approach "Slim Sizing".

*Slim sizing is a natural way to permanently decrease your caloric intake and still consume the things you like.*

Portion control really is diet liberation. The notion that 'bigger is better' has taken over the food industry and this mentality has radiated outward, affecting the size of our pants. We are bombarded with huge, out of control portions that distort our thinking. In order to get our money's worth, or to feel satisfied, we come to expect large portions. Restaurant portions have steadily increased; the average dinner now provides the equivalent of six portions. A study conducted by Pennsylvania State University revealed that the more food we are served, the more we eat, 30% to 50% more in fact. The super sizing of the food industry has caused many of us to suffer from 'portion distortion'. I'll never forget the time I was helping my grandmother move out of her home into a retirement community. I was wrapping up her plates when I asked my mother where her dinner plates where. To my surprise, the plates that I thought were her side plates were in fact her dinner plates. It goes to show that over time, we are super-sizing everything - even our plates!

Here's a fact, no matter what you eat, no matter how healthy it is, no matter what the label says, no matter the quantity of calories it has; if you eat more calories than you burn, you will gain weight. Obvious right? Well, by slim-sizing our plates, and therefore our portions, we are unaware of just how many calories we consume and therefore why it seems difficult to lose or manage weight. Unfortunately, portion sizes have been growing steadily in North America over the last 30 years and expanding portion sizes is the primary reason that we are facing an obesity epidemic. Calories add up quickly when portion sizes are too big. For example, the average bagel in 1970 weighed two to three ounces and contained 230 calories. Today, the average bagel is twice as large and contains about 550 calories. If you eat a larger serving, you will end up eating more calories than your body actually requires. The net result is weight gain due to the excess calories not used. What happens to these extra calories? You guessed it - they are converted and stored as fat. And, as a reminder of what over-eating does to our digestive process, we are left with less energy and less calorie burn because your body is in digestive mode for too long.

Mission Slim Possible is not a diet; it's a life-long path to healthy living and the ideal you. We want to rid our lives of fad diets - these simply restrict the number of calories or types of food you can consume for a finite period of time. But the problem with finite is that once the diet ends, most often, a resumption of the previous way of eating begins, and the weight lost creeps back on. Studies confirm this phenomenon and find diets ineffective for not only the recurrent pre-diet weight gain, but often people will gain additional weight, ending up at a much worse and unhealthy state than when they started.

Portion control is not a diet, but rather, a natural method to control the amount of calories you consume and really need.

With big plates and super-sized servings, it can be very difficult to figure out what an acceptable portion really looks like. If you're wondering how you're supposed to eat 'normal' portions of food in a world of super and mega-sizes, don't despair. You are in control of your portions at home and when dining out. Since it is hard to look at food and know the amount of calories it contains or recognize proper portion size, it is important to adopt some strategies. Even for nutritional professionals, counting calories is a challenge since there are so many variables involved. Being on the Mission Slim Possible Program it is not necessary to count calories but rather keep track of what and how much you have consumed in a day. I don't include calorie counting because, even as a nutritionist, I cannot accurately predict or measure exactly how many calories are in each serving due to the many factors that play a role, not to mention that tracking every morsel of food that enters my body is a daunting task! I don't believe that every little calorie makes a difference - it is portions of food that lead to weight gain.

**Portion control tips to help you on your Mission:**

Now that you know how important it is to pay attention to how much you eat, it is time to apply this knowledge. However, keep in mind that these are basic guidelines. Since adequate portions vary from person to person and day to day, you may have to eat differently. Use visuals, such as some examples given below, to assist you in your ability to associate a standard amount. You can estimate how much to put on your plate or evaluate how much you want to eat from your plate at a restaurant by making these visual assessments, and any uneaten portions can easily be taken home in a doggy bag!

## Eat smaller portions by decreasing the total amount of food:

- Eat the size of a deck of cards for fish, meat and poultry.
- Eat a walnut-size dollop of peanut butter.
- A shot glass full of salad dressing.
- One stamp-size of butter.
- Cereal portions the size of a baseball.
- Rice or pasta the size of one tennis ball.
- Breads, pancakes, or waffles the size of a CD.
- Cheese the amount of four dice.
- Juice the amount of one yogurt container or water it down.

## Use your hand and eye to guesstimate your accurate portion size:

- One finger length for cheese, meat, fish or poultry.
- One layer of your palm or one fistful for mixed nuts.
- Two cupped hands for cereal.
- One rounded handful for cooked pasta.
- One finger tip for butter or oil.

**Tips for when you are at a restaurant -** Plan to say no to the bread right at the start of the meal. Eat to a point of feeling 80% full then stop eating. Ask for half your meal to be packaged up to take home. Ask for your plate to be taken away, physically move it away, or cover your meal with your napkin when you've finished so you don't continue to pick at it. Avoid buffet style anything. If you cannot avoid a buffet, use a small plate and only serve yourself one time. Eat slowly!

## More ideas to help you eat mindfully and control portions:

- Make your kitchen the only eating zone (i.e. avoid eating in front of the television).

- Plan ahead - if you know you eat a lot at certain times of the day, save up some portion of your overall daily intake for that time of the day.

- Recognize if you are eating more because of stress, boredom, procrastination or sadness.

- Avoid missing meals.

- Stop yourself from over-eating.

- If a certain food really is a problem for you, avoid that trigger food.

- Use smaller plates and bowls.

- Avoid buying jumbo bags and boxes of food (studies show we tend to pour more out of bigger boxes than smaller ones).

- Work on seeing food for what it really is (fuel for the body), and eat to sustain the weight you want to be.

- Eat when you are seated and aware.

- Fill up on fresh vegetables and fruit. Start with eating healthy foods when you are starved (studies show people that start with salads eat 12% less calories during that meal).

- Read food labels to understand the actual amount of calories per serving just to get a gauge on what you are really consuming and to determine what your actual serving size should be.

- Avoid second helpings - wait 15-20 minutes first to see if you really need the second helping. Chances are you won't want it.

- Drink water before and after your meal to ease hunger.

- Be cautious with juice drinks (water them down to dilute the calories).

By recognizing portion sizes and using visual comparison or hand measurements, you will become more aware of the amount of food you actually put into your body. You will develop your own internal portion size awareness. The restaurants and manufacturers are not doing it for you, so doing it yourself is important. You can take your knowledge with you wherever you go. No one puts the food in your mouth except you. You decide.

You have control of exactly how much you eat, and therefore you have control over your weight.

**Slim size your meals and portions to help you on your Mission:**

The key to portion control is to slim size your meals. Slim sizing is a natural way to permanently decrease your calories and still consume the things you like. Remember, portion control is diet liberation. Be sure to pick and choose with variety in mind, and don't trade off too much of one food for another without considering calories first. Just having portions in mind could be enough to help you weight balance. If you cut back on your portions, you cut back on calories and so there is no need to diet, to eliminate an entire food group, or to create an imbalance in your body. You want to make great choices while getting the least amount of calories for the most nutrients. As well, select foods that contain the most fiber to feel full and to balance your blood sugar levels. Try to pick the best from each food category; such as the best carbohydrates, the best proteins as well as good quality fats. Don't forget about the vital minerals, vitamins and water.

Be sure to record your food consumption and portion intake into a food journal to keep better track of what you are eating and how much.

If losing weight and eating healthy are two goals you want to work to achieve, then one of the most effective tools you can use is to track your food consumption. The medical community supports this strategy, and I am a firm believer in this too, that one of the best ways to lose weight and keep it off is to simply keep track of the foods you eat. Keeping a food journal reveals eating patterns and allows for a clear indication of amounts. When you have to write down what you're eating and every nibble counts, you might start to have second thoughts about the quality and quantity of what you are putting in your mouth. Furthermore, keeping a food diary has been shown to double your weight loss goals. In one long running study on weight loss conducted by Dr. Jack Hollis, found that by simply writing down the foods you eat, you consume fewer calories and decrease your portions by fifty percent. By keeping track of what you eat, you become aware and mindful of what and how much you eat. You don't have to carry a pen and notepad around where ever you go, simply find a system or program that works for you. Log the type and quantity of foods you consume, and if you can, how you feel when you eat those foods. Perhaps eating a bag of chips made you feel guilty or very thirsty? Perhaps a glass of milk made your gut hurt? By logging your food intake, you can not only measure and become aware of quantity, but the physiological and mental affect food has for you.

There are many ways to do this such as with a journal, a chart, or one of the many applications on our mobile devices that are available to you. My personal favorite is www.myfitnesspal.com. Do your best to record what you are eating and the amount you are eating, being totally honest. Remember your goals. Be aware of 'portion distortion'. Portion control is tough so take one day at a time. Developing size awareness is a learning process; focus on making small changes that you can comfortably live with for life. It really is simple; you want a smaller body, you need to feed a smaller body. If you want a larger body, then you need to feed a larger body. You can adjust your weight by adjusting your portions. As well, one of the most important adjustments you can make is in your attitude. Abandon the 'clean your plate' and 'more is better' syndrome that keeps people from being healthy and slim. In addition to this, eat mindfully and slow down. The more mindful you are, the better you will digest and assimilate the food you eat into your body.

This week will allow you to explore how you can use visualization to drive positive change, both in your weight-balancing approach as well as in your life overall! By creating a picture of your goals in your mind and keeping that image fixed, you have the capability to turn that image into a reality. The only person responsible for your success is you. Group exercise can give you that extra push and motivation to reach your weight balancing goals and keep you on your Mission. By slowing down and eating mindfully, you not only improve digestion you will eat less calories. The key to portion control is to slim size your meals. Slim sizing is a natural way to permanently decrease your calories and still consume the things you like. Remember, portion control is diet liberation. This is the time to let your imagination go crazy. Let yourself dream up a new you and new life for yourself. Stay on your Mission and your outer reality will begin to conform or align with your inner reality.

# STAY ON TARGET

## MY WEEKLY CHECKLIST

- ☑ Use Visualization
- ☑ Paint a clear picture of goal
- ☑ Try group exercise
- ☑ Slow down eating
- ☑ Monitor portions
- ☑ Use your imagination
- ☐
- ☐
- ☐
- ☐
- ☐
- ☐
- ☐
- ☐
- ☐
- ☐
- ☐
- ☐

## MY WEIGHT THIS WEEK:

Began at:_____

Finished at:_____

Total weight loss:_____

## MY MEASUREMENTS THIS WEEK:

### BEGAN AT

Shoulders:_____

Chest:_____

Waist:_____

Hips:_____

### FINISHED AT

Shoulders:_____

Chest:_____

Waist:_____

Hips:_____

### DIFFERENCE/TOTAL INCHES LOST:

Shoulders:_____

Chest:_____

Waist:_____

Hips:_____

What really resonated for me this week?

_____
_____
_____
_____
_____
_____
_____
_____
_____
_____

What worked well for me this week?

_____
_____
_____
_____
_____
_____
_____
_____
_____
_____

# WEEK FOUR

## Psychology Management/Self-Coaching

Define your idea of what slim and healthy is for you. Learn acceptance, believe in your self and notice the pressure around weight balancing decrease!

## Recreation Management

Movement matters. Find every excuse to move. Simple ways to cut calories and increase the use of the calories you do consume.

## Nutrition Management

If you diet now you could end up gaining weight later. Get diet revenge and stop the on and off cycle once and for all. Discover how fat can help you slim down and be healthy.

*"Wanting to be someone else is a waste of the person you are"*

— *Marilyn Monroe*

# — WEEK FOUR —

## Psychology Management/Self-Coaching

Define your idea of what slim and healthy is for you. Learn acceptance, believe in your self and notice the pressure around weight balancing decrease!

Welcome to week four of Mission Slim Possible! This week will allow you to explore how you can use acceptance and belief in yourself to drive positive change, both in your weight-balancing approach as well as in your life overall! If you believe it is possible for you to reach your goal and you can see your success already you will be successful. Many of us are hard on ourselves and don't realize the attention we give the negative energy. This week is all about defining your idea of what slim and healthy is for you. Is it realistic? Is it attainable? Do you really want to be slim? It is time to get real about your weight. Self esteem and confidence in yourself and acceptance is all about how you evaluate yourself. And the fact is that if you don't rate yourself very highly, others won't either and ultimately your day to day actions will not support your goals. Acceptance is a tough one, but we need to start somewhere. This week is two fold, learning what slim and healthy really is for you and learning acceptance to help manifest the belief that you are worth the Mission and can do it.

> *"You can search throughout the entire universe for someone who is more deserving of your love and affection than you are yourself, and that person is not to be found anywhere. You, yourself, as much as anybody in the entire universe, deserves your love and affection."*
> *- Gautama Buddha*

### Define your idea of what slim and healthy is for you:

We live in a society where looks are of utmost importance - there is pressure to achieve 'ideals' of attractiveness. The pressure to be thin, in particular, is at an all time high for women as they compare themselves to models and celebrities in the media. And, this high expectation and comparisons threaten body satisfaction and healthy eating. For the past three decades, women and, increasingly, men have been preoccupied with how they look. Research by Connor-Green, 1998 indicates that up to 88% of women wish to lose weight. Previous research indicates that media, peers and family, along with social comparisons, all may have a serious influence on body dissatisfaction and body esteem.

As Dr. Phil often says, "It is time to get real about your weight". Slim is not a number on your scale and it is not the runway model look. It is time to figure out what is a realistic weight for you and what is really important. Defining your idea will put things into better perspective and help you realize the target of your Mission.

### Slim is: (taken from my clients over the years)

- When you feel you look great (not compared to anyone else).
- When you walk up the stairs easily.
- When your friends say you look great and healthy.
- A weight you can achieve without a big struggle.
- When your clothes fit nicely.
- When crossing your legs doesn't take effort.
- When you feel wonderful to be alive.
- When you are proud with the way you look.
- When you feel sexy.
- When shopping is fun.
- When you feel energized and happy.
- When you are proud to go out and socialize.
- When you are excited to wear jeans.
- When your husband, boyfriend, wife, girlfriend gives you compliments.

### Are you really that bad?

Face a mirror - forget about the media and forget the pressure you put on yourself. Let go of your old notions of slim, instead, see yourself as you really are with lumps, bumps, cellulite and all. Recognize your health and see yourself as strong, energetic, and happy. Recognize your beauty and what you do like about yourself. Focus on what others may compliment you on. Focus on that positive feedback you get that makes you feel good about your self. Are you so bad? Self esteem and confidence in yourself and acceptance is all about how you evaluate yourself. And the fact is that if you don't rate yourself very highly, others won't either and ultimately your day to day actions will not support your goals. How do you feel inside every time you step out of the house? Think about walking in a grocery store or picking up the kids from school and how do you feel about yourself? If it's a bright, cheery day you see outside your door, then go on and enjoy that sunshine. But if it is hard to see that sunshine, it is time to evaluate the relationship you have with yourself. No one but you can make you feel bad! It is time to notice what you have good going for you. Try to remove unrealistic expectations and pressure you might put on yourself. Focus on the positive and take immediate action to get you closer to your target. If somebody were to throw a ball at your head, would you just stand there and let it hit your head or would you try to move aside and let it pass? The choice is in your hands. Even though you may not be feeling that great about your self at this current moment, the complaining and the negativity you give yourself has to stop. It is damaging to your self-esteem and level of acceptance. Accept where you are (without criticizing), evaluate and find what is great about you, then take immediate action to start moving closer to your goals. Make sure your target is a realistic one for you.

If you don't like your current situation, stop complaining and giving it destructive energy. How you react to situations and life is entirely up to you. Acknowledge and move on.


### Believe in yourself and your Mission:

Many of us are hard on ourselves and don't realize the attention we give the negative energy. Every time you look in the mirror and you say, "I look fat," or you say, "I'm not good enough," or "this will never work," you set yourself up to support that thought. This way of thinking inhibits our success with the program. Know that you can do it. If you asked most people how much they would love to complete and reach their goals, they would tell you how amazing that would be. Why do so many people fall short of their weight-loss goals, or any goal for that matter? Simple; they don't believe that they can, so effort and motivation fall short. You are the only one holding you back.

You can complete your goals. Yet until you firmly believe this, stay positive and believe in yourself and target it won't happen. This is one of the major reasons targets and goals need to be realistic. Take the time to visualize your goal and see yourself living your goal. Make sure it is realistic. This will make things more real and help you believe your goals can happen. Reverse or stop negative self talk and criticism that stops belief and halts your progress. Plan to do at least three things that support your goals every day. Say things that help you believe in your self. Take time to notice what is great and already working in your life to help you believe you can achieve great things. This will help you see progress and connect you to the belief it can happen for you. To succeed, we must first believe it is possible that we can reach our goals. Belief comes from realistic expectations, positive self talk and self esteem along with action towards your target.

### Stop comparing yourself and focus on your personal Mission alone:

Though it's been said a million times already, it still holds true that every single individual on this planet is unique - like snowflakes. What matters is not whether you are as good as the rest of the world, but whether you are good at being you. People have different lives and different goals. They all have their successes and failures. Understand that we all are in this together - we are on the same team. Biologically, we are a social species and must learn to accept and be united for the common good.

### Catch the negative critic in you:

We are often so harsh on ourselves, yet most negative thoughts are simply superfluous. It is time to ease up on the pressure you put on yourself. Bring in the new positive voice and become an expert at catching the critic, throw him or her out of your system and bring in a new, more sensitive voice. Simply start thinking good thoughts about yourself. For example, if after you go shopping you are not thrilled with the size of your pants, or hop on the scale and you don't like what it reads, you may begin to berate yourself, but just stop in your tracks, catch that thought, refuse to give it energy and replace it with an effective positive thought. Followed by immediate action towards your target.

### Shift to a place of respect for yourself:

Love yourself because if you don't love and respect yourself, then how can you expect others to respect you? You are amazing, accept yourself, however you are at this moment, and that means physically and mentally. If you are sporting some excess weight at this time, accept it. Endowed with courage? Embrace it! You are special and so respect every aspect of who you are. Because, whoever you are and however you are, there will always be something unique and special in you that nobody else will have. All you have to do is find that out and really love who you are all the time.

## Keep a personal journal along your Mission:

Write something nice about yourself in your journal every day. Whenever you feel down and have low self-confidence or esteem, open up your journal and encourage yourself once again. Try saying three good things about yourself to the mirror each day. If you cannot think of anything to say, think of what a good friend or family member might say about you. Tell yourself you are born a star! Everyone is a star in their own way!

Take time now to think about what is your idea of 'slim'. Is it realistic? See yourself but only better. Have high standards for yourself but keep them realistic. Put this picture into your realistic goals and visions and let it guide and inspire you. By picturing yourself as being realistically slim and healthy, it will make weight management more idealistic, comfortable and realistic. Recognize your goals and decide to love yourself on a deep level during the process; by feeding yourself with positive self-talk, with realistic goals and images, and you will then be that much more equipped to actually achieve what you desire. It is unrealistic expectations that cause you to feel down. The negative self talk and pressure halts your Mission. These high expectations can be dangerous to your psyche. Take the time to evaluate what you are expecting of yourself and recognize if you are being realistic or simply too demanding on yourself. Get an unclouded vision of what you can really achieve, and that can be your goal!

Now that you have a clear image of your desires, allow Mission Slim Possible to be your liberation from diets. Move forward and be happy with your results thus far. Answer these following questions to help you stay positive and desire action to your realistic target.

## Stay positive by answering these reflective questions:

- How can I acknowledge my success?
- What goals have I reached?
- What makes me unique and special?
- What rewards can I give myself?
- What message would I write to myself as an outsider?
- Moving forward, how can I make the remaining weeks on this program more successful for myself?
- What needs to happen?
- What makes me already awesome?
- What do I need to do to reach my goals?

Try the following acceptance affirmations, they may help you stay positive and on target.

Inner love affirmation - As I take a deep breath and my mind becomes quiet, I choose to smile. I begin to hear the gentle voice of my heart. My heart reminds me of its vast reservoirs of loving, kindness and courage that I can draw from as I encounter the challenges of the world. The gentle voice of my heart whispers "I love myself," and it reminds me to see clearly the loving, wonderful person that I am. I am on the same team as my mind and body, I choose to love and work with my whole being. Deep in the stillness, I see clearly there is no need to insult, deny or be cruel to myself. I am a happy, loving and a wonderful person that makes a difference in people's lives. I make others smile and I deserve to love myself, to be kind to myself and be patient with myself. I love myself, I love myself, I love myself!

Be yourself affirmation - Today, I resolve to appreciate the unique loving person that I am. I choose to be the person I desire to be. I resolve to follow my inner voice and intuition; to be me wholeheartedly. My quiet mind and open heart prepare the ground for my very existence. My presence assures me there is no need to worry about performing or doing the right thing or being someone I am not for others. Just by being myself, others will love me and I will love myself more. I am a great person. I make others smile, laugh, and they enjoy my company. By just being myself, I follow my inner voice and I bring out the best in myself and others. By being me, I am happy. This presence allows my caring being to always be authentic and healing. Today, I take courage and strength to just be myself and remove the worry or pressure to be something I am not. I feel freedom in the security of being myself. Today, I practice presence as I care for myself and those around me. I am myself, as I listen, laugh, cry, share joys and sorrows. I am me, one-hundred percent, and others will love me for it. I am real and I feel a sense of simplicity. This simplicity guides me and keeps me happy. I am happy to be me, happy to be myself, and happy others love me for me!

*"For once, you believed in yourself. You believed you were beautiful and so did the rest of the world." - Sarah Dessen*

Define what your idea of slim and healthy is for you. Question if it is a realistic goal for your self. Change your thinking from being hurtful or critical of yourself to acceptance and self-appreciation. By moving out of the negative critical mode and into learning acceptance mode, you can better believe in your self and pressure around weight balancing will decrease! The path towards your target on your Mission, when filled with acceptance, self love and action, will be a positive one. This week, I suggest you take courage and strength in being yourself, acknowledge where you are at, stay positive and take immediate action towards your realistic target.

### It's time for self-coaching and inner reflection:

Take time to answer and work through these questions in your journal to help keep you focused and on a clear path towards your goals. By taking action you will bring your goals into your life. These self-coaching questions will help clarify what you need to have accomplished this week.

### Self-Coaching Questions

- What needs to happen each day this week?
- What are my priorities this week?
- How will these action steps help me get closer to my goals?
- In the next week my complete focus will be on?
- My direction is clear to me because...?
- I am willing to commit to...?
- What might success look like to me for this week?
- What resonated and stood out to me from the program and what impact will it have on me this week?
- I deserve this because...?
- I am thrilled with myself because…?
- Why is it important for me to take action and follow my goals this week?

# — NOTES —

*"If you don't move your body, your brain thinks you're dead. Movement of the body will not only clear out the "sludge," but will also give you more energy"*

— *Sylvia Brown*

# — WEEK FOUR —

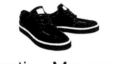

## Recreation Management

Movement matters. Find every excuse to move. Simple ways to cut calories and increase the use of your calories.

**Movement makes a big difference along your Mission:**

We need to move our bodies every day, period. Running, walking, spinning, biking, whatever your choice is, you've got to do some sort of movement every day. The more you move, the easier it will be to keep your weight down, stay healthy, and you will feel better and more alive! But, sometimes we need that little extra reason to get us out there. Feeling in control and at peace with your body is foundational to feeling in control and at peace in your life. Exercise is for everybody! Free yourself from what weighs you down. Get rid of the excess baggage in your life and find strength inside you never knew you had.

Want to hear something that may shock you? Your body actually likes exercise. Huh? "Not my body," you might say. But think again. Your body may not be used to exercise, but given the chance, your body will amaze you with responsiveness. We are designed to move. Every little bit of movement makes a difference in our ability to manage our weight. Learn to move regularly and lose body fat, and you will be rewarded with a firm sense of personal accomplishment, a tighter stronger, leaner body, and a confident glow that lets you know you can do anything you put your mind to...anything! It's also great for clearing your head and for feeling more grounded and centered. You are your own work of art!

Feeling slim and toned is empowering in and of itself. Staying active at the gym, using exercise machines, participating in group exercise, and even a walking or running regimen are all great ways to become fit, increase stamina, gain strength and burn calories. But they aren't the only ways to get moving. To overcome the inertia of a sedentary lifestyle and begin to enjoy the sensation of moving your muscles, a more gradual approach, which increases your desire to move, might be the best long-term way to begin. The founder of Canada's largest and best known gym chain, GoodLife Fitness, David Patchell-Evans, says the principles of fitness and exercise is like brushing your teeth. One of the main reasons people don't exercise are because they are intimidated. 'Patch' says, "All it takes is three times a week. Think of it like brushing your teeth. Imagine if you had to brush harder and better every time – people would probably quit brushing altogether. Like so many things in life, sometimes success is about just showing up." I love this mentality and completely agree. Choose to show up this week and stay on your Mission with consistency. You can do it. One way to start is to identify those parts of your regular day that you consider "inactive," and then take steps to reduce them by replacing them with some kind of movement. You can do this easily by moving in a way that doesn't feel like a workout, or by approaching your workout time in a different frame of mind.

**Try to incorporate movement into your life as often as possible:**

Is life conspiring to keep you away from the gym this week? Fear not! The following tips will help keep you strong and slender, whether you're stuck at home, in the office or in the car. Even if you are a dedicated gym enthusiast, you can squeeze some or all of these additional forms of movement into your day. This extra movement will improve circulation and be a great way to burn extra calories. Additionally, taking breaks from your computer, or other sedentary tasks, to stretch, move and strengthen, will benefit not only your body, but your mind and spirit as well. There are many ways you can incorporate movement into life, this is just a starting list. Use your imagination to get movement into your life.

1. Take the stairs.
2. Park your car farther away and walk.
3. On buses, subways, or when someone is driving you, get off before your destination and walk part of your way.
4. Take a walk during your coffee break.
5. Start a movement hour where you work.
6. Garden.
7. While watching television, do a burst of exercises while the commercials are on.
8. Put on some music and dance. Or, go out dancing. Take dance lessons!

9. Buy an exercise video and then use it. Go on YouTube and get inspired.

10. Have sex frequently.

11. Rake the leaves into piles and jump into them, then rake them again.

12. Mow the lawn with a hand-mower.

13. Shovel the snow from your driveway and then do your neighbour's driveway too.

14. Vacuum and clean the entire house.

15. Clean out the closets or the garage.

16. Help a friend move.

17. Wash all your windows.

18. Jump rope or jog while watching television.

19. If you work in an office, make phone calls standing up.

20. Play games like catch, Frisbee, tag or touch football with the kids.

21. Play miniature golf.

22. If you golf, don't use a golf cart.

23. Join an organized sport like tennis, basketball, volleyball or badminton. Go bowling.

24. Wash your car and vacuum it out.

25. Walk while you talk on the phone.

26. Walk the malls, or go power-shopping.

27. Take your dog for a hike on the trails.

28. Scrub the kitchen and bathroom by hand.

29. Plan to meet a friend weekly to shoot some hoops.

30. Take the kids (or grandkids) to the park and push them on the swings.

31. Go snowboarding or skiing.

32. Try snow-shoeing or cross-country skiing.

33. Pick your own fruits and vegetables on U-Pick farms.

34. Keep weights out in your house and every time you pass do some exercises.

35. Find a pool and splash around like a kid.

36. Try rollerblading.

37. Paint a room.

38. Go backpacking.

39. Try paddle boarding, canoeing or kayaking.

40. Re-arrange the furniture in your house.

41. Hold a family picnic and have relay or three-legged potato sack races, tug-of-war, and play badminton.

42. Try walking in the river.

43. Ride a bike.

44. If you are close to your school, walk with your kids instead of driving them.

Fitness can be fun. It's all about the way you think about it and your attitude. It simply involves moving and being active. Imagine for a moment that you suddenly lost movement in your legs - all you would want is to be able to walk and run again, so don't take your ability to move for granted. Instead get yourself thinking that exercise and movement is a good thing and enjoyable. If you do it regularly, not only will you get more energy, core strength and muscle tone, but you will also have fun. "When activities and healthy lifestyle choices are incorporated into daily living, staying active becomes second nature," says Orthopedic Surgeon and AAOS spokesperson, John Purvis, M.D. It can be as simple as making a list of fun, active things that you like to do. Then begin to make those things part of everyday living. Every little bit of movement burns calories, improves circulation and makes a difference in your natural weight balancing attempts.

*"I've been on a diet for two weeks and all I've lost is fourteen days."*

— Totie Fields

# — WEEK FOUR —

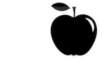

## Nutrition Management

If you diet now you could end up gaining weight later. Get diet revenge and stop the on and off cycle once and for all. Discover how fat can help you slim down and be healthy.

### What is a diet?

We don't often think about what the word "diet" really means. For most of us, it conjures up thoughts of the measures people take to lose weight. For others, the word diet may signify "healthy" as many manufacturers use this word to indicate that something is supposedly healthier. But the word "diet" itself really means what we eat. We seem to hear about people going on diets, but your diet really is what you eat day to day. However, most people refer to a diet as a temporary plan that one might go on to lose weight. So, for this section, a diet or dieting is defined as a period of time where one restricts the amount of calories consumed and where meals usually follow some obscure and strict protocol. This restrictive type diet is the type of diet that we are referring to, and does not work for balancing weight. Dieting is a method of losing weight that will work in the short term but is usually followed by disappointment and rebound weight gain. This mentality sets you up for failure and a sense of weakness. Many times these diets have certain gimmicks or themes, such as eating foods by percentage of macronutrients (fats, proteins, carbohydrates), or some ask you to eliminate a food group altogether. Some diets are downright unhealthy and even dangerous. The main issue with diets, as referred to for the purpose of this program, is that they simply don't work. People find that they can't stick to a diet for a long period of time because the program is too costly, restrictive, too hard, too complicated, or too inconvenient to maintain. Not to mention, we are hard-wired to like foods that are high in fat and carbohydrates, so we simply don't have the willpower.

### How to get diet revenge!

Your body needs a certain number of calories each day just to maintain normal metabolic function. Your lungs, brain, heart, muscles, digestive system, nervous system and cardiovascular system all require calories to work properly. Acquiring the proper number of nutritiously dense calories each day will ensure that you are functioning at your best and you will have a proper ratio of fat to lean muscle. However, when you diet, the net result is a change in your body composition because diets are, more often than not, much too low in calories. If you drastically reduce your caloric intake too quickly and abruptly, your body will switch into starvation mode and begin to conserve energy by down regulating the number of calories burned at rest. While on a diet, your body will utilize the quickest form of energy - from your muscle - before it uses energy from fat. So, in actuality, the end result when you diet you decrease the amount of lean muscle you have and you end up having more fat stores. On a diet you end up not requiring as many calories to sustain yourself and these excess calories get stored as fat, not the body-changing composition you were going for I bet! As you deplete your muscle mass, your caloric requirements reduce, but what is often seen with individuals who stop dieting and resume a "normal" caloric load, the body will store all of these extra calories as fat if it does not require the excess amount of calories. Since the body composition has changed and the amount of energy or calories decreases, the body therefore, stores the excess calories as fat. The body will not use the "extra" calories consumed post-diet and convert them back to lean muscle - nor will fat automatically convert to lean muscle. Since you need lean muscle to stay lean and healthy, you need to consume healthy calories in order to fuel your body and keep it running efficiently. The more muscle you have, the more calories you burn, the more food you can eat, and the more likely your body will use up your fat stores.

### Don't jump on the 'low-carb' bandwagon & get diet revenge!

The percentage of people that re-gain the weight they've lost while on most diets is high, but it's even higher with low-carb, high protein diets.

## Long term negative implications of low-carb diets:

A recent trend in the weight-loss world is the low-carb (keto-genic) diet. The main goal of low-carb diets is to lose weight quickly by eliminating, or drastically reducing carbohydrates. This particular diet does seem to work well for many people initially, but if you're concerned about long-term health and sustained weight loss, it might not be the way to go. The thought process behind low-carb weight loss is this: starve your body of one kind of energy (carbohydrates) so that it immediately burns another kind of energy (fat). This makes sense in an elementary sort of way, but your organs don't necessarily appreciate the simplicity of the logic. On a cellular level, your body only knows that it is getting lots and lots of fat to burn, but your cells need fat, protein, and carbohydrates in order to function proper-ly and keep your organs performing optimally. When you eliminate carbohydrates from your diet, you're also eliminating fiber, and as you know, you need fiber to keep your intestinal tract working properly in order to rid your body of waste.

### Depletion of muscle stores & fatigue:

There is more, because the preferred form of energy - carbohy-drates - aren't readily available, your body has to go to Plan B - take it from your muscles and liver in the form of glycogen (the storage form of glucose). When you deplete glycogen stores, you dehydrate your body, which causes a significant drop on the weight scale initially. However, this deceptive drop is, in fact, primarily due to dehydration and muscle loss (this is why this diet has become so popular!). More-over, the depletion of muscle glycogen will lead to muscle atrophy (loss of muscle). This happens because muscle glycogen (broken down to glucose) is the fuel of choice for the muscle while moving. Without glycogen readily available to your muscles, the muscle fibers contract less - both at rest and while moving. Depletion of muscle glycogen causes fatigue and less energy to exercise and move. This lack of energy and decreased movement leads to muscle loss and the inability to maintain adequate muscle tone. When good quality carbohydrates are not available, the muscle is literally used up for fuel because there is easily accessible muscle protein for direct metabolism. The body converts the stored muscle glycogen to glucose for fuel. Research indicates that muscle fatigue increases in almost direct proportion to the rate of depletion of muscle glycogen. With this drop, individuals don't feel energetic and exercise and move less, which is not good for caloric expenditure and basal metabolic rate (metabolism). So much like the paragraph before, this diet does not work and the net result is a change once again in your body composition. Metabolism happens in the muscle. Less muscle and muscle tone means a slower metabolism which means fewer calories burned throughout the day.

Low fiber & unhealthy:

Further to that the low-carb diet lacks in a sufficient amount of your daily fiber requirements. You must obtain fiber from plant-based and whole grain based foods - you cannot get this from meat products. A deficiency in fiber could increases your risk for cancers of the digestive track because transit time (the rate a which food is passed through your body) is lengthened. It is also linked to cardiovascular disease due to decreasing the health benefits of fiber and the effect it has on fat and cholesterol. It also puts you at a higher risk for constipation and other bowel disorders. Fiber also helps regulate the absorption of glucose into the blood and therefore keeps blood sugar levels consistent. Low-carb diets are simply not healthy as they lack in fiber and lack sufficient quantities of the many nutrients, phytonutrients, and antioxidants found in the foods you are asked to eliminate from your diet, such as fruits, vegetables, legumes, and whole grains - all of which are necessary for good health and weight management. In fact, you need these nutrients even more when you are trying to off-set a nutrient deficit which ends in weight gain. Can it get worse? What else happens on a low-carb diet? Your muscles and skin begin to lack in tone and become saggy. Loose skin and muscles don't look good. You begin to lose a healthy, vibrant look (even if you've also lost fat). A sunken, unhealthy disposition is the ultimate appearance of high protein, low-carb diets.

There are some not so good carbohydrates choices:

Some proponents of low-carb diets recommend avoiding carbohydrates such as bread, pasta, potatoes, carrots, etc., because of they are high on the glycemic index - causing a sharp rise in insulin levels. Certain carbohydrates have always been, and will always be the bad guys: candy, cookies, baked goods with refined sugar, sugared drinks, processed, or refined white breads, pastas, and rice, as well as any foods with refined sugar. These are not good for your health or weight management. However, carbohydrates such as fruits, vegetables, legumes, whole grain breads, whole grain pastas, and brown rice are good for health and weight loss. Just as with proteins and fats, these carbohydrates should be eaten in moderation. Large volumes of any proteins, fats or carbohydrates are not conducive to weight-loss and health. A balance of every food category is essential for overall health and weight maintenance.

High protein can be high in bad fat:

High protein diets means you are eating too much of the wrong fats, and eating too much of the wrong fat is just not healthy. Meat proteins contains, fat and cholesterol along with potential antibiotics and growth hormones. I know you've heard of people whose blood levels of cholesterol and triglycerides have decreased while on a low-carb, high protein diet. This often happens with any weight loss, but it doesn't continue when the diet you are on is high in fat. There are literally reams of research over decades that indicate an increase in consumption of animal products and/or saturated fat leads to increased incidence of heart disease, strokes, gall stones, kidney stones, arthritic symptoms, and certain cancers to name a few. Fat is certainly necessary, and desirable in your diet, but the source should be mostly healthy fats and consumed in moderation. It is common for people to see high protein diets working and people often state, "it must work - people are losing weight".

### The net results of low-carb, high protein diet can be:

- You lose muscle mass. With that comes a slower metabolism, which also means fewer calories being burned.
- A loss of muscle during the process of losing weight which changes body composition and leads to future weight gain.
- The healthy fluids lost during the low carb diet you end up re-gaining
- It's difficult to maintain that type of restriction diet long-term.
- Long-term healthy lifestyle has been challenged.
- You decrease fiber and precious nutrient levels in your body compromising health.
- You decrease your energy levels and thus burn less calories.

### Get diet revenge & avoid the fat free diet craze!

In addition to the low-carb craze, the fat-free craze has also brainwashed our society over the past couple of decades. Let's begin with a very clear fact: fat-free diets will not make you fat free. People figure that if they eat foods that say they are "fat-free", they will not get fat. Yes, you can lose fat while restricting fat intake, however, we need some fat to survive, feel satisfied, and regulate absorption of food. Fat in foods slow down stomach emptying and help increase the feelings of fullness and satiety after a meal. Not feeling full is one of the major reasons diets end in failure. Grocery stores line their shelves with products that state "fat-free", "lite", "light", and "low-fat", and these words are effective marketing tools for those seeking less fat in their diet. It would follow that if you wish to lose weight, you would consume low-fat or fat-free products, however, this logic is flawed. What is often overlooked is the fact that these foods have added sugars, salts or artificial chemicals to make up for the loss of taste by removing fat. All these additions are usually very unhealthy and result in other health problems in addition to weight gain.

### Fat is actually good for our health!

Fats are actually an important part of your diet and are essential for your body to function optimally. Every cell is made up of proteins and fatty acids. It is these fatty acids that are essential for our bodies to function properly. In terms of weight loss, fats make us feel satisfied and content with what we eat. Fats also add flavor, it slows the absorption of sugar into the body, and provides sustained and prolonged energy. Good quality fats are essential to maximizing your weight loss and to helping you feel great. They are the key to regulating blood sugar levels, cravings, hunger, and the mobility of fat out of the body.

Also, fats remove toxins from the body by stimulating bile. This process works as bile emulsifies fat, which then binds to toxins (unwanted chemicals in the body), and removes them, as well as any excess fat, from the body.

### Knowing the different types of fats:

Saturated fats are saturated with carbon molecules and they are hard at room temperature. They are found in most animal products such as steak, hamburgers, butter, and cheese. These fats will harden your arteries after a while, as they are hard in nature. These fats should be eaten in moderation, both in terms of your overall health, but in particular, if you are managing or trying to lose weight, the consumption of these fats will be stored in your body until it gets the good quality fats it is seeking. So, again, eating saturated fats should always be done in moderation!

Trans-fats are man-made fats. This includes deep fried foods, rancid oils, and margarine. They are toxic to the body because our bodies lack the ability to metabolize this type of fat. The result of consuming trans-fats is free radical damage, and your body responds by making cholesterol to counter the effects. Trans fats are unsaturated fats which are uncommon in nature but can be created artificially. The American Heart Foundation states that Trans fats raise your bad (LDL) cholesterol levels and lower your good (HDL) cholesterol levels. Eating trans fats increases your risk of developing heart disease and stroke. It's also associated with a higher risk of developing type 2 diabetes. Before 1990, very little was known about how trans fat can harm your health. In the 1990s, research began identifying the adverse health effects of trans fats. Trans fats can be found in many foods – but especially in fried foods like French fries and doughnuts, and baked goods including pastries, pie crusts, biscuits, pizza dough, cookies, crackers, and stick margarines and shortenings.

Essential Fatty Acids are the good quality 'fat' guys. EFAs are essential to get from our food as we do not produce these naturally. EFAs break down into omega-3 fatty acids and omega-6 fatty acids. EFAs are particularly important because they help with feeling satisfied, they support your nervous system, they improve your immune system, they make your hair and skin vibrant and they will also mobilize unwanted fat stores out of your body. We need fat for many health reasons but we also need proper fats for weight management. Since every cell in the body is made with these fatty acids, your body will begin to function better and will use the fat you consume in all areas of your body leaving none for storage. What a bonus when you try to squeeze into your sexy jeans and there is no squeezing required! It is important to know which fats are the good fats, such as essential fatty acids, as these fats will make you healthier, more radiant and slimmer!

| **Sources of EFAs** | | |
|---|---|---|
| Eggs | NutsSeeds | Olive Oil |
| Coconut Oil | Flax seed oil | Borage oil |
| Safflower oil | Fish | |

**Get diet revenge with healthy balanced eating:**

The good news is getting all the macro-nutrients is the best realistic diet. This means getting protein, fats and carbohydrates into all your meals, everyday! People that are losing fat on low-carb, high protein diets, are doing so because they are eating fewer calories - that's the bottom line. There is no magic - the same can be done on a healthy diet that is more sustainable and without elimination of any of the essential macronutrients. By eating the way nature intended us to eat, you will be healthier, and greatly increase your chances of managing and keeping weight off. Your natural ability to balance your body is called homeostasis; this process is far stronger than any willpower! In other words, you have a strong mechanism built in you to make sure things stay balanced. If you throw this off, your body will do what it takes to bring things back into balance. To be truly healthy, you need to consume foods from a large array of food categories, and this includes the whole grain breads (rye, rice, spelt) and pastas (rice, kamut, spelt), which as you now know, are big no-no's for a low-carb diet. As is the case with most quick fixes, though, the shortsightedness of it all makes it too good to be true. While your stomach feels full on a high protein diet, you're still essentially starving yourself.

### Slow, steady, and consistent effort towards your Mission, will get you to your target:

You have seen the magical pills and the diets that guarantee "RESULTS FAST!" But, once the pills have run out and the diet ends, the empty bottles and gadgets are put aside and you body begins to return to where it started and guess what? The fat returns. The body is a complete, intelligent system that is not fooled by diets. You cannot deprive it and expect it to keep functioning optimally. Thankfully, it doesn't have to be this unhappy ending. You can easily manage your weight naturally with consistent effort without sacrificing your health. Keep away from extremes, and remember the most effective strategy may not be the quick, easy way, but rather the consistent, realistic natural way nature intended for us!

## Focus on the following:

- Steady, healthy whole food choices.
- High nutrient saturation and low calories.
- High fiber foods from natural sources.
- Good quality fats.
- Healthy food choices from every food category.
- Smaller meals with good portion control.
- Build muscles.
- Exercise consistently.
- Consistent effort towards your goals.
- Slow and steady wins the race.

## Nutrition summary

- Diets do not work. They merely change your body composition and lead to future weight struggles.
- The key to prevent yourself from going on a restriction diet of any kind is to think about achievable, realistic changes you can sustain.
- You must exercise and keep your muscle mass up by doing weight-bearing exercises. Keep your muscles for strong metabolism.
- Avoid fat-free or fad diets of any kind.
- Consume good quality fats to manage hunger and fat metabolism.
- Choose a natural, realistic approach to manage your weight.

This week is all about defining your idea of what slim and healthy is for you. Is it realistic? Is it attainable? Do you really want to be slim? It is time to get real about your weight. Self esteem and confidence in yourself and acceptance is all about how you evaluate yourself. It is time to figure out what is a realistic weight for you and what is really important. Defining your idea will put things into better perspective and help you realize the target of your Mission. Movement matters in your life. There are many ways you can incorporate movement into your life, the key is to just get started. Movement, getting tone and fitness can all help with confidence levels and setting realistic targets. If you diet now you could end up gaining weight later. Get diet revenge and stop the on and off cycle once and for all. Even though you may not be feeling that great about your self, when you are further away from your target, the complaining and the negativity you give yourself has to stop. It is damaging to your self-esteem and level of acceptance. Accept where you are (without criticizing), evaluate and find what is great about you, then take immediate action to start moving closer to your goals. Making sure your target is a realistic one for you.

# STAY ON TARGET

## MY WEEKLY CHECKLIST

- [x] Define your idea of slim
- [x] Put things in perspective
- [x] Find new ways to be active
- [x] Find ways to accept yourself
- [ ] _____
- [ ] _____
- [ ] _____
- [ ] _____
- [ ] _____
- [ ] _____
- [ ] _____
- [ ] _____
- [ ] _____
- [ ] _____
- [ ] _____
- [ ] _____
- [ ] _____
- [ ] _____

## MY WEIGHT THIS WEEK:

Began at:_____

Finished at:_____

Total weight loss:_____

## MY MEASUREMENTS THIS WEEK:

### BEGAN AT

Shoulders:_____

Chest:_____

Waist:_____

Hips:_____

### FINISHED AT

Shoulders:_____

Chest:_____

Waist:_____

Hips:_____

### DIFFERENCE/TOTAL INCHES LOST:

Shoulders:_____

Chest:_____

Waist:_____

Hips:_____

What really resonated for me this week?

_____
_____
_____
_____
_____
_____
_____
_____
_____
_____

What worked well for me this week?

_____
_____
_____
_____
_____
_____
_____
_____
_____
_____
_____

# WEEK
# FIVE

## Psychology Management/Self-Coaching

Discover the motivation to stay focused on your target. Taking action is the only way you can reach your personal goals.

## Recreation Management

Building strong lean muscle mass will help you naturally manage your weight, boost your metabolism and help you look amazing. There is benefit in a good night sleep.

## Nutrition Management

A strong metabolism can naturally manage your weight. You can boost your metabolism with certain food choices and methods of eating.

*"Stay focused, go after your dreams, and keep moving towards your goals."*

*— LL Cool J*

# — WEEK FIVE —

## Psychology Management/Self- Coaching

Discover the motivation to stay focused on your target
and goals. Taking action is the only way you can reach
your personal goals

Welcome to week five of Mission Slim Possible! This week will allow you to explore how you can discover your motivation to help you stay focused and take action. This week we will create a clear target so you can take immediate action on your Mission to reach your goal. If you want something bad enough and your motivation is strong, you can find ways to make it happen for you! Focused motivation can feed your desire and make positive change, both in your weight-balancing approach as well as in your life overall! You are very important and deserve the outcome you seek. Don't hold yourself back - let nothing stand in your way, not even your weight. Set your target strong this week and shoot the arrow continuously towards your target!

*"If it is important to you, you will find a way. If not, you'll find an excuse." - Magic Johnson*

### Goal setting and having clear targets are essential to your success:

Goal setting and having a target to shoot towards, is an extremely important tool for personal development and self-change. By setting goals we give ourselves a target to shoot for and we are better able to measure our progress along the way. You might have noticed on the cover of this book, I have a bow and arrow, symbolizing being on a Mission with a clear target in mind. I have always said to my clients, "Desires without a target and action, is like day dreaming." Imagine what happens when you shoot an arrow without a target, goals need to be narrowed down with precision, focus, and clarity.

### Why having clear goals & specific targets are important:

- Goals keep us moving forward and motivate us.
- They are the foundation to success.
- Goals bring us focus: Imagine shooting an arrow without a target
- Goals allow us to measure our progress: Goals give endpoint so you know the steps you need to take to get you there.
- Goals give us barriers and limits: They help us stay away from distractions and keep us focused towards our target.

- Goals help you overcome procrastination: Goals give us responsibility and ownership for our life.
- Goals give us motivation: In the end one of the main purposes of goal setting is to provide motivation and drive.
- Goals give us Determination: Supply fuel to push forward towards something.

### How to set realistic targets for yourself:

- Write your target down: Makes your target more real and powerful, committed and reflective.
- Set Short term Milestones: Far out of reach targets end up in procrastination. Set mini milestones to help stay on track and feel successful.
- Be target specific: The more specific the better, the more motivation, and focus.
- Measure your actions as well as your progress: Action measuring can keep you motivated. For example; instead of measuring pounds lost, measure the amount of cardio done.
- Start with just one target: Focus on 1-3 things at a time
- Schedule in time for your target: If you don't make time you'll never reach your goals. Allocate time each day or week towards your target.
- Set targets you actually want to achieve: Not because you think you should! If your husband wants you to lose weight and you are happy with where you are then that target is not realistic for you. Pick targets you want to achieve for yourself.

## Why sometimes we miss our target:

- Setting process targets, rather than results targets: support the thing you want to create not the process to get there.

- Setting ideals not visions as goals: Ideals are should goals and visions are want goals. "It would be nice to weigh 115 like I was when I was 20", is an ideal goal.

- Setting targets that are too vague and general: Such as "be healthy", be very specific what you want to achieve.

- Setting realistic targets instead of stretch goals: Stretch goals are goals that are not realistic or even achievable.

- Setting targets that are not grounded in reality: You must clearly know your destination and your starting point. Ground your vision into reality.

- Setting targets that are ego driven: Make sure goals are not just about you, but rather about results you can create. What is your primary focus? Getting specific on heart felt results goals are more powerful. For example, completing this book was a specific target for me. My target was about: helping millions of people reach their fullest weight management potential, sharing the secret about natural weight-loss, giving people the tools to apply a healthy realistic approach. My reason for reaching this target, was very specific and clear for me and Not ego Driven at all.

- Setting targets but not taking appropriate action: I'm sure you've heard many versions of "A vision without action is like day-dreaming"; you must act on your goals.

## How to make your arrow hit the target effectively:

- Target setting is a powerful tool for creating results and generating success.

- Set clear and compelling results focused targets. See and feel your results as if it were fully completed.

- Make sure your target come from heartfelt desires, not demands.

- Make your target and visions as clear, compelling, and detailed as you can. Include specific success a criteria. Establish standards of measurement with which you can measure your progress, and know when you're done. For example, how many pounds can you lose each week. Or how much time you spend walking per day.

- Set "stretch" goals that far exceed your current capacity. Set your standards high! Big targets stir our souls, and draw our best out of us. Set realistic targets only in the context of, and in support of your big, super, stretch goals. That'll provide you maximum motivational power.

- Ground your target in reality. This provides you a solid platform on which to take action. Targets need to be realistic for you.

- Be wary of your ego. It's OK to want the rewards that come with successfully creating results, but remember it's the result that comes first, not your ego.

- Take action. Learn from both your mistakes and successes. Build the momentum and take appropriate immediate action.

If you set targets using these principles, you will be able to rise above your current situation and obstacles, learn what you need to know and do, and make consistent progress toward realizing your dreams. Only you create the life you want for yourself.

**Now, take action toward your goals:**

Jump into life with both feet, take action and get the results you are looking for! No one is going to do it for you. Jump into life and do exactly what you want to do and be who you desire to be. Take back control of your life by making the decisions and choices your need to make to reach your targets. Nothing can stand in your way unless you let it. Participate in your life instead of waiting for another day. Decide what you want and go for it whole-heartedly. You will be amazed with how often you get exactly what you desire. Stay focused on your goals and desires, if anything gets in your way, overcome the barrier. You are very important and deserve the outcome you seek. Don't hold yourself back - let nothing stand in your way, not even your weight. Put on that bikini regardless of how you think you look, have fun and enjoy your life. Do not wait for the 'perfect' body, as you will miss all the fun. So delve into your life and truly enjoy what it has to offer you! The more powerfully driven you are to take immediate action, the more likely you will reach your target. When the pull towards your target is strong and you keep taking action everyday the distance between your target and where you are currently decreases. If you want to live a life of purpose, fulfillment and passion, it's up to you to take back your power, and take action today towards your goals. It's time to stop whining, generating excuses and making imaginary obstacles. You can follow your passion if you will make the decision to take action. Reclaim your power and take back responsibility, because you realize that you alone are responsible for your success. Suspend any disbelief and believe that you can create a life where you are proud of what you look and feel like. Slow and steady wins the race. Be consistent with your action and watch your target get closer. Live here and now. Be happy now in the process towards your target. Follow your desire and passion, but make sure it's something you enjoy doing in the process.

### Connect to where you find motivation?

Two of the biggest problems people often have with achieving their goals are getting started and staying motivated to stick with their goals. But, believe it or not, two of the biggest motivators to get people going are typically fear and hitting rock bottom - not the ideal places to start. I know that I have had moments in my life, where it felt so terrible and the situation was a great kick in the butt to get me motivated. Ideally, though, we don't want you to have to hit rock bottom. So, here are some better places to find the motivation to get you started and keep you going.

**Change your perspective:** Shift your thinking to what you do want for yourself from what you don't want. Instead of, "I don't want to be fat" you can say, "I want to be slim and fit."

**Identify very clearly what you want:** Paint that picture of what you desire. Keep it handy. Connect to your target daily, hourly, and every minute if you can.

**Set your targets:** Put a date to your goals in bold letters on the calendar. Commit to your program or target and make it a priority.

**Set realistic mini targets:** Large targets can feel daunting and over-whelming. Those are the stretch goals we talked about earlier. Stick to monthly, weekly, daily and even hourly goals. What are some action steps to get you to your goals?

**Think about making it fun and full of options:** Look for as many options you can think of for your target. Have fun brainstorming all the ways you can reach your target. Chances are there are more options than you realize.

**Make it become a habit:** Repeat, repeat and repeat again those actions that work you towards your target. I heard somewhere that it takes 21 days to form a new habit. Commit to something and see if it can become a habit for you. Chances are if it makes you feel good and aligns you with your target, it will become a habit for you.

**Listen to your inner voice:** Follow what is really important to you. Strive to your target for this reason alone, It is important to you.

**Reach out to others for support:** Such as a friend, family member or a spouse to help you positively with your target. You probably have more resources and support than you realize.

**Build into you what you need to reach your goals:** If you build your goals into your life, you are more likely to stay motivated. Remember, if you want a body like an athlete, you have to act like an athlete. If you want to weigh 120 pounds you have to eat and exercise like a 120 pound person.

**Look for potential excuses:** Isolate those barriers or potential excuses and come up with solutions around them. Do this before the barriers show up so you already are equipped with a solution.

**Write it down:** There's something official and meaningful about seeing your ideas in black and white. It is a concrete commitment when you write it down. Writing down your goals will make it official, like a certificate for yourself legitimizing your goals.

**Spread the word:** Don't be afraid to tell people what you are working towards. You won't get off too easy if you tell people what you are striving towards. Sometimes, though, silence and steady progress towards your target works for some people. You decide.

**Be flexible:** It is nice to have goals and think about them often, but be flexible if you stray off them momentarily. Don't give up or beat yourself up because you couldn't set aside that hour one morning to exercise. The key is to treat your targets like very important events and add it to your daily schedule, but be flexible.

**Practice forgiveness:** Don't despair if you miss a workout on your path towards your weight balancing goals because of a busy schedule. The important thing is to get back up and work towards your goals as soon as you can.

Do you remember the New Year's resolutions you set at the beginning of this year? What are they? How are you doing so far? If you are like most people, chances are you've long abandoned those goals. Don't get discouraged though, because target setting works and rarely fails. The only reason why goals aren't reached is due to giving up. Only you can decide what is important to you, and only you can achieve your target. But with these few motivational steps the sky is the limit. You can achieve your goals no matter what they are. It's all a matter of staying focused.

### How to stay focused on your target and keep your eye on the prize!

**Concentrate:** Don't spread yourself too thin. Pick one to three goals that are most important to you, and stick to them. Don't think about those other desires until these ones are achieved. Laser like focus can allow you to make progress!

**Create a vision board:** (As mentioned earlier in this book) A vision board is a collage of pictures and images that represent your goals and dreams. Creating and viewing this board helps you to visualize your end goal more clearly, which inevitably inspires and motivates you to take consistent action towards your target.

**Create milestones:** If you just set one huge goal it can feel like your goal is far away and this can lead to procrastination. It is helpful to break down big goals into smaller goals.

**Create a plan:** If you have worked out a plan for attaining your target, it becomes so much easier to stick to the plan. Following the action plans you have created day after day will get you to your goals. Create that action plan right after you choose a target. The more action you take towards your target, the target actually starts moving closer to you as well.

**Track your success:** It's important to track your results and your accomplishments. On Mission Slim Possible you want to track your measurements, your weight and your mini successes along the way. These little success reminders can help you stay focused on your target, and make you feel like you really are making a difference.

**Journal your goal pursuit:** Having a private journal to document your goal pursuit can be a therapeutic experience. A lot of times we abandon our goals because we get frustrated mid way. When you write your thoughts, successes and remind yourself of why your goals are important, you get clarity and a renewal of motivation.

**Learn to say "no" if you need to:** Do you often put your goals on the back burner to help or support other people? It's okay to do that once or twice, but if this is consistent in your life, then you will not reach what is important to you. You can't put your goals on hold for others, you need to say "no" sometimes and you may find a bigger reward when you attain your goals.

**Be clear on why your target is important to you:** If you give up on your target half way, ask yourself how important was that goal to you? You need to get serious about your goals and not give up on them if they are truly important for you. Constantly remind yourself why your goal is important to you and how you will feel when you accomplish your target.

## The courage to succeed affirmation (Read aloud to yourself):

It takes just as much energy to succeed as it does to fail. There is just as much work and energy and just as much difficulty to having success as there is to have failure. I realize that I must work actively to stay slim and healthy or waste energy by gaining weight and jeopardizing my health. I choose to be proactive on my Mission. The exact same effort is involved in both cases, but directed differently. When I put no effort or energy into achieving my goals, I spend enormous energy resisting what comes naturally. Humans naturally strive to achieve and experience success in all of their undertakings. It takes a great deal of effort to stop short of accomplishment. I choose to succeed. I choose to be the best version of myself. I would much rather put my effort into success then waste my energy in failure. Therefore, success calls for a certain degree of courage, the courage to be aware of the decisions and obstacles that we put on our path to success. This exercise requires enormous discipline and precision. But when we set out to take stock of our limitations, and work to better ourselves, we open our minds to success. Success requires another form of courage; the courage to live a greater and more demanding life and to go beyond the personal limitations we have known so far. Today, I choose to take immediate action on my Mission. Today, I make positive use of my courage and I move forward to greet the future. To succeed!

*Take charge of your life...*

### It's time for self-coaching and inner reflection:

Take time to answer and work through these questions in your journal to help keep you focused and on a clear path towards your goals. By taking action you will bring your goals into your life. These self-coaching questions will help clarify what you need to have accomplished this week.

### Self-Coaching Questions

- What needs to happen each day this week?
- What are my priorities this week?
- How will these action steps help me get closer to my goals?
- In the next week my complete focus will be on?
- My direction is clear to me because...?
- I am willing to commit to...?
- What might success look like to me for this week?
- What resonated and stood out to me from the program and what impact will it have on me this week?
- I deserve this because...?
- I am thrilled with myself because…?
- Why is it important for me to take action and follow my goals this week?

# — NOTES —

*"Work out not to look good, but to make others look bad."*

— *Anonymous*

# — WEEK FIVE —

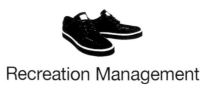

## Recreation Management

Building strong lean muscle mass will help you naturally manage your weight, boost your metabolism and help you look amazing. There is benefit in a good night's sleep.

**Exercise and movement:**

Being active has a major influence on metabolism. The speed at which your body metabolizes food into energy depends on two key factors: how many calories you consume and how many calories you burn. Exercise increases your requirement for energy and keeps your metabolism active in order to meet the increased need. When you exercise, your body increases the speed at which you burn calories and therefore, speeds up the metabolism. When you stop exercising your metabolism is still revved, so it continues to burn calories at an increased rate for some time. Exercise also sets off the release of endorphins (feel good hormones), which make you feel euphoric and happy. So, get moving, keep moving and you will see the benefits to your health and how effectively you can manage your weight.

### Muscle can almost act like magic helping you get closer to your target :

Is it true that the more muscle you have, the higher your metabolism will be? Yes! Muscle burns more calories than fat stores do, so when one increases their lean muscle mass, they also naturally raise their metabolism. When you have more muscle, you require more energy production and thus you speed up your metabolism. The more muscle you have, the more calories you burn, the more food you can eat, and the more likely you will use up your fat stores just to sustain yourself. There is nothing other than your muscles that will make your body burn more calories while you are at rest, even while you sleep. Strength training exercises, such as lifting weights and resistance training, are especially effective for building muscles. Strength training increases your body's lean muscle tissue and increases the rate at which your body burns calories. Lean muscles require many calories just to exist. When you increase your lean muscle mass, you fire up your metabolism as a result!

The best way to build muscle naturally is through short, intense workouts that use resistance of some sort. This type of muscle stimulation creates growth. If you want bigger muscles you must provide stimulus to them in the forum of regular workouts. When you lift weights or use the body's own resistance and do the movement slowly you will build muscle mass. Fast lifting causes you to use momentum, rather than recruiting the muscle. Don't swing the weight, as this stops the isolated muscle from working to maximum effort. Try this: Do a biceps curl slowly and controlled as a full extension down and then curl up versus quick, abrupt movements. Slow is always harder because the isolated muscle is working. Resistance, or strength training, involves activities that use weights, machines, resistance bands or even body weight to work your muscles properly. There are a ton of sites on the internet that provide free workout routines involving resistance training. This can be extremely helpful in achieving a healthier body. Training with weights is typically associated with athletes who bulk up and have excessively big muscles and it can deter some (particularly women) to use weights in fear of getting big, masculine muscles. But, in fact, resistance training is simply about increasing the strength of the body, not always its size. Resistance training basically strengthens the muscles, and leans the body of fat stores. One of the best things about resistance training is that it can be done with little to no expensive equipment and does not require a large amount of space. Doing push-ups is one good example. You can do it just about anywhere there is enough space for you to move. In addition to an increase in bone density and strength, muscles will grow stronger and become more developed as you progress. Using and increasing muscle mass (even a little bit) will increase the energy that is required by your body, even at rest. This also increases the energy needed by your body during activities. The more muscle, the more energy is required to be broken down to supply your body with usable energy in order to function properly. This translates to more fat calories and fat being burned each minute. Thus, with the decrease in body fat, you can expect the tone of your body to improve and you will become a lean, mean, fat busting machine and did I mention sexy? See, muscle is magic! There is a cute anonymous writer quote poster going around these days, it says, "Skinny people may look good in clothes, but fit people look good naked." I couldn't agree more. Muscle IS tone.

**You can build muscle at home with these home workout ideas:**

Home muscle-building workouts offer convenience, time saving, and privacy. If for whatever reason you can't make it to the gym, you can build muscle right at home. Building muscle with home workouts is attainable and requires a set of free-weights used three times per week for half an hour to an hour each session. I highly recommend the muscle burn workout based on strength trainer, Steve Shaw. His principle is that muscles respond differently to different repetition ranges. For each workout, choose your muscle group and two to three exercises for each muscle group. Then, perform at least two "power sets" using sufficient weight to tire the muscles after three to five repetitions. Next, perform at least two "muscle sets" using enough weight to tire the muscles in six to twelve repetitions. Finally, perform at least one "burn set" using enough weight to tire the muscles in fifteen to twenty repetitions. Rest only long enough to regain strength, and then continue performing reps in this set until you reach a total of about forty reps each exercise. Shaw recommends working chest, biceps, buttocks and abdomen on day one; quadriceps, hamstrings, calves and abdomen on day two; and shoulders, triceps, back and abdomen on day three.

Feeling confused or unsure? There are numerous resources online, at the library, and at the gym of sample exercises for each muscle group. Once you tire of the basic recommendations, be sure to change up the two to three exercises per muscle group with any new exercise. Be sure to practice proper form and ask a trainer or someone familiar with proper form if you are unsure. This is beyond the scope of this book, however, do, do your research and find a good muscle building program for yourself.

**Sample week of muscle workout:**

You can vary the days, times and exercises, but follow the basic training principle for great results. The following website is a great resource for all exercises and videos on execution: www.bodybuilding. com. Some exercises won't follow the set principle, in which case, try to do about 40 repetitions.

|  | LOAD/RESISTANCE | REPETITIONS (REPS) |
|---|---|---|
| Power Set | Super heavy for you | 3 to 5 reps |
| Muscle Set | Medium heavy for you | 6 to 12 reps |
| Burn Set | Lighter for you (still challenging at 15-20 reps) | 15 to 20 reps |

| | MUSCLE GROUP | EXERCISE |
|---|---|---|
| Monday | Chest<br>Biceps<br>Buttocks/Gluts<br>Abdominals | butterfly<br>Bench press<br>Hammer Curl<br>Bar curl<br>Glut kickbacks<br>Bridge<br>Bicycle |
| Wednesday | Quadriceps<br>Hamstrings<br>Calves<br>Abdominals | Lunges<br>bench jump<br>Dead lift<br>Wall run<br>Calf raises<br>Seated raise<br>Heel raise roll-over |
| Friday | Shoulders<br>Triceps<br>Back<br>Abdominals | Side raise, over head<br>Bench dips, skull<br>crush<br>Bent row, pullover<br>Elbow to knee, leg<br>pulls |

Maureen Hagen, VP of Operation, GoodLife Fitness, has been one of my long time mentors and inspiration in the fitness and wellness field. She has wonderful resources for everything fitness. She has authored numerous books and articles along with continuous blogs to help you stay motivated to get fit. I highly recommend her Newbody Workout For Women- 6 Weeks to a Fit and Fabulous New You. Dec 29, 2009. Penguin Canada. It is the perfect program to help you get in shape and maintain a lean, strong body—for the rest of your life.

*"The nicest thing for me is sleep, and then at least I can dream."*
*- Marilyn Monroe*

### Sleep can renew your spirit, bring you energy and support your metabolism:

Sleep makes you feel better, but its importance goes far beyond just boosting your mood and banishing dark circles under your eyes. Lack of sleep is actually not good for our weight management Mission. Sleep deprivation sends the signal to your body to eat in order to increase your energy, thus resulting in consuming excess calories. When you are tired, your brain thinks it is hungry and needs energy from food. Getting adequate sleep is a key part to a healthy lifestyle, and can benefit, your heart, mind, metabolsim and weight (because when you are tired, you burn fewer calories). Sleep researchers have discovered the health implications associated with sleep deprivation, these include:

- Intense sugar cravings.
- The inability to feel full after eating plenty of food.
- Impulsive eating and compulsive overeating.

- Decrease in lean muscle tissue.
- Impaired ability to obtain energy from carbohydrates.
- A decrease in physical activity.

### Can more sleep really help control weight?

While doctors have long known that many hormones are affected by sleep, David Rapoprot, MD, says it wasn't until recently that a correlation between sleep and appetite was revealed. The hormones, leptin and ghrelin, both influence our appetite: leptin tells us we are full and ghrelin tells us we are hungry. And, the production of these hormones seems to be influenced by how much or how little sleep we obtain. Studies revealed that after participants were sleep deprived, their leptin levels dropped and their ghrelin levels went up. In other words, being sleep deprived increases the production of the hormone that tells you you're hungry. Ghrelin works under the principal that, when the body is tired, it will send a signal to your brain to say "feed me", in order to gain energy.

Many of us sacrifice sleep in order to get more things done. There are so many more important things to do then waste time sleeping, right? There's an inherent problem with this logic, however. The quantity and quality of your sleep directly affects the quality of your waking life, including mental sharpness, metabolism, physical vitality, and even your weight. These studies and the negative affect of sleep deprivation might help you rethink this mentality. So, depriving your body of some required z's, is actually counter-productive to your wake time. You will slow your productivity, your physiological efficiency and sacrifice your health.

In order to keep your body running at its best, manage your weight, and provide sixteen hours of sustained wakefulness, you need between seven to nine hours of sleep each night. No other activity delivers so many benefits with so little effort! Make bedtime an appointment with yourself. Start a bedtime ritual and make a restful routine. Be sure to avoid sugar and caffeine before bed. Take a bath or warm shower as they tend to relax your muscles and calm your mind by raising your body temperature slightly. Getting seven to nine hours of good quality sleep will increase your energy and metabolism! The good news is that you don't have to choose between a slim body and productivity. As you start getting the sleep you need, your energy, metabolism and efficiency will go up and your ability to better manage food cravings will also improve. If fact, you're likely to find that you are actually more productive during the day when you are not skimping on your shut-eye.

*"While weight loss is important, what's more important is the quality of food you put in your body. Food is information that quickly changes your metabolism and genes."*

— Mark Hyman

# — WEEK FIVE —

## Nutrition Management

Your metabolism naturally manages your weight, but we cannot blame metabolism for gaining weight! You can support the metabolism with certain food choices, body composition and methods of eating.

### What is metabolism?

Metabolism, commonly defined by dieticians as the chemical processes that occur within a living organism in order to maintain life, or more specifically, the chemical changes in living cells by which energy is provided for vital processes and activities and new material is assimilated. Metabolism converts the fuel in the food we eat into energy needed to power everything we do, from moving to thinking and growing. Every time you swallow a bite of sandwich or slurp a smoothie, your body works hard to process the nutrients you've eaten. Long after the dishes are cleared and the food is digested, the nutrients you've taken in become the building blocks and fuel needed by your body. Metabolism keeps your body systems going at an efficient rate by providing the cells with the required nutrients it needs, whether it comes from food intake, fat stores or glycogen stores in the liver. Metabolism, simply put is the rate we change our food into fuel. Excuse me while we get scientific for a bit, specific proteins in the body control the chemical reactions of metabolism, and each chemical reaction is coordinated with other body functions. In fact, thousands of metabolic reactions happen at the same time, all regulated by the body, to keep our cells healthy and working. A faster, productive metabolism will be efficient and will provide plenty of energy to the body. A slower metabolism will decrease the rate at which your body can function because you rely on the energy from your metabolism to be active. This needed energy is not only used for physical expenditure, but also for its internal jobs, such as breathing, digestion, heart beats, and electrical impulses to name a few. Metabolism is responsible for all action in the body!

*"What you want is to rev up your metabolism so that you are burning fat and calories, not preserving fat and calories."*
*- Kathy Freston*

**Metabolism and how it relates to weight management:**

You have probably heard people blame their weight on a slow metabolism, but what does that mean? Is metabolism really the culprit? And if so, is it possible to rev up your metabolism to burn more calories? While it is true that metabolism is linked to weight, it may not be in the way that you expect. In fact, contrary to popular belief, a slow metabolism is rarely the cause of excess weight gain. Although your metabolism influences your body's basic energy needs, it's your food and beverage intake, as well as your physical activity that ultimately determine how much you weigh. The bottom line is; a calorie is a unit that measures how much energy a particular food provides. If you provide your body with more calories that you can burn off, the excess is stored as fat. Not a great result when you are trying to lose weight. The number of calories that you may burn in a day is directly related to how active you are, the amount of fat and muscle you have, as well as your basal metabolic rate (BMR). This is a measure of the rate at which you burn those calories at rest. This is where your metabolism plays a role. When a person has a slow BMR, they burn fewer calories at rest versus a person with an average BMR, who will burn more calories at rest, when both are consuming the same amount of food. Every person's metabolism works in a unique way, determined by several hormones produced by the endocrine system. Thyroxine, a hormone produced and released by the thyroid gland, plays a key role in determining how fast or slow the metobolic chemical reactions occur in a person's body. Although your BMR is something you're born with, you are able to alter this to an extent simply by changing your lifestyle. When you exercise, you burn more calories, but you are also becoming more physically fit, and by that, you are speeding up your BMR. And, as you increase your fitness, increase your muscle mass and reduce the amount of fat stores, you will increase your BMR, thereby creating a positive cycle of burning more calories than storing and thus losing weight. So your metabolism can be influenced to a certain degree.

Enhance the natural process of metabolism with eating and drinking water!

**Eat at regular intervals:**

When you miss meals, your body interprets this as a possible fast. Taking all possible measures to keep you alive and anticipating starvation, your body starts to conserve fuel, burning fat and calories more slowly. Then when you do eat, your body stores everything in case of a future famine. The body goes into a conservation mode, reserving its energy while burning fat and calories at a slower rate. Metabolism slows to an almost halt in response to starvation, even with just one missed meal. When you eat less or go into starvation, you slow all your processes down, your body starts to move at a snail's pace and your energy greatly decreases. To further our understanding of how metabolism plays a role, it's helpful to know how our body generates and stores energy. I introduced to you the basic concept of BMR, but metabolism is a complex process. There are two types of metabolism - one that creates and stores energy for the body, and one that releases energy into the body. Both work simultaneously and function depending on the needs of your body at any particular time. For example, when you eat, your body typically will go into constructive metabolism (anabolism) and store energy in the form of carbohydrates, protein and fat. Destructive metabolism (catabolism) is the process of utilizing these energy stores for all body functions. So, when you consume more calories than you burn, the net-result is an excess storage of energy in the form of fat - and in many cases ends in weight gain.

Countless studies show that people who eat meals on a regular and consistent basis are much more successful at losing weight and keeping the weight off than those who skip meals. Eating meals at regular intervals prevents over-eating and incorrect portions at future meals by avoiding the feeling of 'starvation' and a ravenous appetite. Believe it or not, eating more frequently can actually cause you to lose weight. As ironic as that sounds, when you eat more frequently you burn more calories.

The key to weight-loss is to fire up your metabolism by eating more often than you were, but not more food than what you were eating.

When you diet, you typically drop your caloric load to below what your body is used to by skipping meals. But, this tricks the body into thinking it should store and conserve energy. If your body thinks that energy supplies are limited, then it will slow and conserve where necessary. This manifests itself in poor physical energy levels, less strength, and a lifeless disposition. The body begins to draw inward for focus on the important and basic life processes such as heating and breathing. Instead, your body is happy to receive food at regular intervals. When you eat smaller meals at regular intervals you can shrink the size of your stomach and after a while, you will feel full eating less food. The decrease in the amount of food and calories eaten helps reduce weight.

### Thyroid supportive nutrients:

Your thyroid gland is located in the throat area and it is responsible, in part, for regulating your metabolism by the secretion of certain hormones. When there is an imbalance in the secretion of these hormones, your metabolism is affected. Hypothyroidism, for example, is an underactive thyroid. Typical signs include lack of energy and weight gain (among other things). Many times the body suffers from an underactive thyroid that is subclinical or not at a stage where the condition can be treated with medication. I highly recommend that you have your thyroid checked regularly by your medical doctor. Since the thyroid regulates metabolism, it is important that you provide the essential nutrients it needs to function. The thyroid functions mostly on a mineral called iodine. A diet rich in iodine has been shown to help regulate your thyroid. Just by adding iodine sources to your diet, you will assist your thyroid to function optimally. Food choices that contain iodine are found in the sea. Sea vegetables are your best sources of iodine. They include: kelp, dulse, nori, vegetarian sushi, miso soups, sea salt (edible and/or non edible for your bath) and fish. Other foods include: beans, water herb teas, olive oil, flaxseed oil, safflower oil, almonds, walnuts, low-fat meat, rice, and vegetables. Coconut oil contains lauric acid, which stimulates thyroid function, increasing metabolism and weight-loss. I recommend using culinary grade coconut oil when baking and cooking. Dulse, a red algae, is rich in iron and loaded with essential minerals, B vitamins, C, A, and E vitamins and is particularly high in iodine, a metabolic mineral very important for the thyroid gland and brain function. In addition, dulse has the highest frequency of all essential minerals, acts as a controller for calcium metabolism, and protects the brain by destroying toxins in the blood before they pass through the blood-brain barrier. Dulse can be purchased in a powder form and added to your favorite smoothie. Meat sources of iodine include seafood such as bass, cod, halibut, perch, pike, red snapper, shad, sole, sturgeon, swordfish, tilefish, rainbow trout, and yellowtail. Consuming these foods when you suspect a sluggish thyroid may help support this system and therefore help with weight balancing.

**Eat carbohydrates with a low glycemic index measurement:**

Research demonstrates very clearly that whole grains, fruits, vegetables and beans are all beneficial for supporting your metabolism, for weight loss as well as toward the prevention of type 2 diabetes, colon cancer and constipation, because these foods provide clean, usable energy. Say good-bye to refined grains, such as many breads, pasta, cookies and cakes, which cause most people to over-secrete insulin. As part of the constructive metabolic process, insulin is secreted from the pancreas to facilitate the uptake of glucose from the bloodstream into the cells. Too much insulin in response to an excess amount of glucose in the blood, leads to an imbalance of the metabolic process. Remember to choose whole grain carbohydrate sources. Breads are a big part of many of our diets, so choose those made with spelt, rye or rice flours (to name a few).

**Eat the right amount of protein:**

Protein is very important in supporting metabolism and weight-loss because it helps to build lean muscle, which helps burn calories quickly. The more muscle you have, the more calories you burn, the more food you can eat, and the more you are likely to use up fat stores. The hormone, glucagon, is released in response to dietary protein, such as those found in eggs, cheese, lean meats, chicken, fish, and protein powder. Glucagon signals fat cells to release fat into the blood, thereby promoting its use. In other words, more fat is burned and more weight is lost when you eat protein.

**Get your green tea:**

Instead of your morning coffee, choose green tea. Green tea has proven to have many health benefits, from helping fight diseases, to aiding in weight balancing. Many various studies have shown that catechins, the antioxidants in green tea, help increase fat burning. Research also shows that green tea may lower blood sugar levels by inhibiting enzymes that allow the absorption of starches, and it may reduce the absorptions of fat from the intestine.

**Consume good quality fat:**

Fats are important for regulating metabolism because they slow the digestion of carbohydrates and allow for sustained long-term energy, keeping your body alive and active longer and as a result and allowing you to burn more calories.

To support your metabolism you need to eat food from all food groups. You need to choose the best foods in these categories to prevent cravings and overeating, and most importantly, you need all food groups at regular intervals to enhance your body's ability to bolster energy and burn calories.

*"There are only three things women need in life: food, water, and compliments". - Chris Rock*

**Water and metabolism:**

Water supports your metabolism, helps with purification, and naturally balances your weight.

The human body is composed of approximately 70% water. In

fact, the body's water supply is responsible for, and involved in, nearly every bodily process, including digestion, absorption, circulation, and excretion. Every cell is filled with water and every chemical reaction relies on water. This includes the essential chemical reactions that take place so that your body can produce energy, allowing you to be active, burn calories, and have an effective running metabolism. Drinking water is one of the easiest efforts you can incorporate into your weight balancing efforts and maintenance plan. Water is calorie free. Think about it, unlike saying no to eating that tempting cheese cake at a party or going to boot camp class once or twice a week, making sure you are drinking enough water requires very little willpower and determination. There's no excuse for not drinking water, and if you're having troubles finding a way to fit your recommended eight glasses a day into your schedule, it's an easy fix when you know all the benefits of drinking water. Here are some great benefits of staying properly hydrated so that you can lose weight and help manage your weight long-term.

Drinking water makes you feel full and gives you a sense of satisfaction. You could mistake thirst for hunger, and overeat.

It's important to know that when you are thirsty, you are already at the point of dehydration. And, being dehydrated can lead you to eat more than you need. Did you know that often when you feel hungry, you're actually just thirsty? Our mind tends to confuse hunger and thirst. When your body needs water, the brain sends the same signal as hunger, often leading to eating instead of drinking water. When you drink water and are properly hydrated, you fill your stomach to avoid this confusion in signaling, and therefore will feel satisfied. You will eat less, and you tend not to over-eat. Consuming less food means less caloric intake resulting in weight-loss or maintenance. When you find yourself hungry at odd times of the day, reach for a glass of water before grabbing food. If you really are hungry, you can still eat a snack afterwards. If feelings of hunger do go away after drinking your water, you just saved yourself the calories by not eating what your body didn't really need. It is recommended that you drink a glass of water before going to any social events, because doing so will help prevent you from over-eating the unlimited array of snacks and food likely to be there. Drinking water can buy you some time to assess your hunger and help you make better choices. So next time you're about to enter a party or situation that might have unhealthy food choices, take time to finish off your water bottle.

## Water is essential for weight management and your overall health

When you're properly hydrated, you have improved blood flow, properly regulated metabolism and as a result you are far more energized (conversely, dehydration slows your blood flow and makes you tired). With proper blood flow, nutrients from the blood (such as glucose and oxygen), provide energy to your cells at an efficient rate, as well as pumping those nutrients throughout your body, allowing your body to work at its optimum. As a matter of fact, your metabolism will slow to conserve energy when you have not had enough water to drink, as your organs can't and won't function as efficiently. In addition, with proper hydration, you flush toxins and fat out of your body, which is essential to good health and weight management. It makes sense that water contributes to your body's ability to burn calories since it's involved in almost all of your bodily processes. Your body needs adequate amounts, particularly during exercise, to prevent dehydration and keep the fat burning process working optimally. To keep the body functioning properly, it is essential to drink at least eight, 8-ounce glasses of quality water each day. While the body can survive without food for about five weeks, the body cannot survive without water for longer than five days. Water can help fire up your metabolism and shed pounds. Drinking ice cold water first thing in the morning is an easy way to support your metabolism and start getting your water intake. Your body will have to warm up the water entering your system, which takes energy. It is a simple step to add into your daily routine that can certainly contribute your good health and Natural Weight Balancing. Another great benefit of staying hydrated is that it helps keep your joints lubricated, which is very important for daily functioning and injury prevention. What's the secret to a clear complexion, youthful radiant skin, healthy lean body, unshakeable energy and a strong constitution? Water, so drink up! Water is essential. We simply cannot live without it. Staying hydrated all the time is vital to your weight balancing efforts and to keep your body working at its best!

### Tips to increase your water and stay hydrated:

- Replace calorie laden beverages with water and drink a glass before meals to help you feel fuller.
- Drinking more water helps support your metabolism.
- Water boosts your energy levels. If you feel drained, get a pick-me-up with water.
- Water helps the blood transport oxygen and other essential nutrients to your cells.
- Staying hydrated keeps your heart pumping and the blood flowing throughout your body. When you're dehydrated, you heart has to work hard to do this.
- Lower stress with water - 85% of your brain tissue is water.

If you're dehydrated, both your body and your mind will be stressed. To keep stress levels down, keep a glass of water at your desk or carry a bottle and sip regularly.

- If you feel thirsty, you're already a little dehydrated.
- Build muscle tone with water. Drinking water helps prevent muscles cramping and lubricates joints in your body.
- When you are well hydrated you can exercise longer and stronger without "hitting the wall."
- Nourish your skin. Fine lines and wrinkles are deeper when you're dehydrated. Drinking water hydrates skin cells and plumps them up, making your face look younger. Water is nature's own beauty cream.
- Water flushes out impurities, improves circulation and blood flow, leaving your face clean, clear and glowing.
- Water helps keep you regular. Along with fiber, water is essential for good digestion. Water helps dissolve waste particles and passes them smoothly through your digestive tract.
- If you're dehydrated, your body absorbs all the water, leaving your bowels dry and more difficult to pass.
- Water can help dilute urine and prevent kidney stones by diluting salts and minerals.

**Metabolism support summary:**

- Don't diet.
- Avoid skipping meals.
- Eat at regular intervals.
- Choose a diet rich in the best carbohydrates.
- Eat good quality protein to support muscle.
- Eat a diet rich in good quality fats.

- Eat foods containing iodine (like dulse).
- Get enough sleep.
- Find ways to be more active.
- Incorporate muscle building in your exercise routine.
- Exercise to burn calories and feel great.
- Drink plenty of water.

## Week Five Final Motivation

This week is all about goal setting and having a target to shoot towards. It is an extremely important tool for personal development and self-change. This week we will create a clear target so you can take immediate action on your Mission to reach your goal. If you want something bad enough and your motivation is strong, you can find ways to make it happen for you! Focused motivation can feed your desire and make positive change, both in your weight-balancing approach as well as in your life overall! Two of the biggest problems people often have with achieving their goals are getting started and staying motivated to stick with their goals. Building strong lean muscle mass, eating foods, drinking water and getting the proper amount of sleep, you will naturally manage your weight, boost your metabolism and it will help you look amazing.

# STAY ON TARGET

## MY WEEKLY CHECKLIST

- [x] Set goals
- [x] Be clear on target
- [x] Create action plan
- [x] Connect to your motivation
- [x] Build lean muscle mass
- [x] Get good sleep
- [x] Drink lots of water
- [ ] _____
- [ ] _____
- [ ] _____
- [ ] _____
- [ ] _____
- [ ] _____
- [ ] _____
- [ ] _____
- [ ] _____

## MY WEIGHT THIS WEEK:

Began at:_____

Finished at:_____

Total weight loss:_____

## MY MEASUREMENTS THIS WEEK:

### BEGAN AT

Shoulders:_____

Chest:_____

Waist:_____

Hips:_____

### FINISHED AT

Shoulders:_____

Chest:_____

Waist:_____

Hips:_____

### DIFFERENCE/TOTAL INCHES LOST:

Shoulders:_____

Chest:_____

Waist:_____

Hips:_____

What really resonated for me this week?

_____
_____
_____
_____
_____
_____
_____
_____
_____
_____

What worked well for me this week?

_____
_____
_____
_____
_____
_____
_____
_____
_____
_____
_____

# WEEK
# SIX

# Psychology Management/Self-Coaching

Stress and its impact on your Mission! Defeat and manage stress with optimism and positive thinking.

## Recreation Management

Yoga and meditation are fantastic for stress management, optimism and can help you on your Mission!
How yoga helps reduce anxiety, reduce pessimism and manage stress.

## Nutrition Management

Get diet revenge and combat stress with nutrition. Understanding the link between stress and weight management.

"The greatest weapon against stress
is our ability to choose one thought over
the other."

- William James

# — WEEK SIX —

## Psychology Management/Self- Coaching

Stress and its impact on your Mission! Defeat and manage stress with optimism and positive thinking.

Welcome to week six of Mission Slim Possible! This week will allow you to explore how you can use optimism, positive thinking and good nutrition to help manage stress and drive positive change, both in your weight-balancing approach as well as in your life over-all. Stress has an impact on your Mission and could move you off your target. Yoga is a fantastic discipline that is helpful with con-necting to your Mission and a form of stress management. Your life is already stressful without having to worry about what goes into your mouth. However, what you eat and how you eat it can contribute to your ability to cope with the stress in your life.

## Understanding stress:

Modern life is full of deadlines and demands. For many people, stress is so common that it becomes a way of life. With the plethora of responsibilities mounting on your plate you can literally feel like your life is OUT OF CONTROL! Guess what? You have a lot more control than you may think; you are in fact in control of your life and you can decrease stress! I often say in my yoga classes, "stress is something that is out there, it is how you interpret the event that makes it stressful." This simple realization is all about taking charge of your thoughts, your emotions, your food intake, your environment and the way you deal with problems.

The ultimate goal to manage stress is to balance your life, your time for work, relationships, relaxation, and fun; plus have the resilience to hold up under pressure and meet challenges!

## What is stress?

Stress isn't always bad. In small doses, it can help you perform under pressure and motivate you to do your best at a task. But when you're constantly running in this emergency mode, your mind and body can pay the price. If you frequently find yourself feeling frazzled and overwhelmed, it's time to take action and bring your nervous system back into balance. Stress is actually meant to protect you and be a good thing. Moderate amounts of stress could actually be healthy for motivation.

When you perceive a threat, your nervous system responds by releasing a rush of stress hormones, including adrenaline and cortisol. These hormones rouse the body for emergency action. Your heart pounds faster, muscles tighten, blood pressure rises, breath quickens, and your senses become sharper. These physical changes increase your strength and stamina, increase your reaction time, and enhance your focus – preparing you to either fight or flee from the danger at hand. Stress is a normal physical response to events that make you feel threatened, or upset your balance in some way. When you sense danger – whether it's real or imagined – the body's defenses kick into gear, this is an automatic process known as the "fight-or-flight" reaction, or the stress response. The stress response is the body's way of protecting you. When working properly, it helps you stay focused, energetic, and alert. In emergency situations, stress can save your life – giving you extra strength to defend yourself or spurring you to press on the brakes to avoid an accident, for example. The stress response also helps you rise to meet challenges and deadlines. Stress is what keeps you on your toes during a presentation at work, sharpens your concentration when you're playing a badminton game, or drives you to study for an exam when you'd rather be watching television. But beyond a certain point, stress stops being helpful and starts causing damage to your health, your mood, your productivity, your relationships, and your quality of life.

### Effects of chronic stress:

The body doesn't distinguish between physical and psychological threats. When you're stressed over a busy schedule, an argument with a friend, a traffic jam, or monthly bills, your body reacts just as strongly as if you were facing a life-or-death situation. If you have a lot of responsibilities and worries, your emergency stress response may be "on" the majority of the time. The more your body's stress system is activated, the easier it is to turn on and the harder it is to shut off. Long-term exposure to stress can lead to serious health problems. Chronic stress disrupts nearly every system in your body. It can raise blood pressure, suppress the immune system, increase the risk of heart attack and stroke, contribute to infertility, and speed up the aging process. Long-term stress can even rewire the brain, leaving you more vulnerable to anxiety and depression.

**First it is good to identify the sources of stress in your life:**

Stress management starts with identifying the sources of stress in your life. This isn't as easy as it sounds. Your true sources of stress aren't always obvious, and it's easy to overlook your own stress-inducing thoughts, feelings, and behaviors. Sure, you may know that you're constantly worried about managing your weight. But maybe it's your procrastination, avoidance, and/or denial rather than the actual weight issues that lead to stress.

### Common external causes of stress

- Major life changes
- Work
- Relationship difficulties
- Financial problems
- Being too busy
- Children and family

### Common internal causes of stress

Not all stress is caused by external factors. Stress can also be self-generated:

- Inability to accept uncertainty
- Pessimism
- Negative self-talk

- Unrealistic expectations, perfectionism
- Personal pressure put on oneself

To identify your true sources of stress you need to look closely at your habits, attitude, and excuses:

- Do you explain away stress as temporary ("I just have a million things going on right now") even though you can't remember the last time you took a breather?
- Do you define stress as an integral part of your work or home life ("Things are always crazy around here") or as a part of your personality ("I have a lot of stress, that's all").
- Do you blame your stress on other people or outside events, or view it as entirely normal? ("You kids drive me nuts and stress me out.")

**Start a journal to keep track of your stress:**

Until you accept responsibility for the role you play in creating or maintaining the stress in your life, your stress level will remain outside of your control. A stress journal can help you identify the regular stressors in your life and the way you deal with them. Each time you feel stress, keep track of it in your journal. As you keep a daily log, you will begin to recognize patterns and common themes. Write down:

- What caused your stress? (make a guess if you're unclear)
- How did you feel - both physically and emotionally?
- How did you act in response?
- What was your behavior like?
- What did you do to make yourself feel better?
- What did you think to make yourself feel better?

**Easy strategies to deal and cope with stress in your life:**

Managing stress is all about taking action and personal responsibility: taking charge of your thoughts, your emotions, your time, your environment, and the way you respond with problems. Stress management is about avoiding unnecessary stress, changing the situation if you can, positively adapt to the situation, accept things that you can't change, take on a healthy lifestyle and get plenty of sleep. Further to that, yoga and meditation are great ways to de-stress and put things into perspective.

**Stress management tips:**

- Avoid what does not need to be stressful. Learn to say "no", and know your limits. Avoid people and situations that stress you out. Take control of the people and things around you. Avoid topics and conversation that gets you heated. Scale back the amount of things you plan into your day. You may be surprised, however, by the number of stressors in your life that can be eliminated.

- Change your situation. If you can't avoid certain situations you can try to change or alter it. Talk it through and express your feelings. Be willing to work with people to compromise. Be direct when you need to be. Managing your time will ease stress. Being early for things, instead of pressing the clock time and time again, can help you stay calm. Decide what you can do to change things so the problem doesn't present itself in the future.

- Positively adapt to the situation, if you can't change the stressor, you can change or adapt yourself. By changing your expectations and attitude you can reframe the problems, look at the big picture and adjust your standards.

- Focus on the positive. When stress is getting you down, take a moment to reflect on all the things you appreciate in your life, including your own positive qualities and gifts. How you think can have a profound effect on your emotional and physical state. Each time you think a negative thought about yourself, your body reacts as if it were in a tension-filled situation. . Eliminate words such as "always," "never," "should," and "must." These are telltale marks of self-defeating thoughts. Think sunny thoughts!

- Accept the things you can't change. Some stress is unavoidable. Acceptance may be difficult, but don't try to control the uncontrollable. Try to look at the stressors as opportunities for personal growth. Share feelings and learn to forgive and let go. Free yourself from negative energy by forgiving and moving on.

- Make time to relax and have some fun. Include rest and relaxation in your daily schedule. This is your time to take a break from all of your responsibilities to recharge your batteries. Spend time with positive people who enhance your life. Make time for leisure activities that bring you joy, whether it be biking, playing the piano, or working on your garden. Have fun and laugh often. You can control your stress levels with relaxation techniques like yoga. There is more on this in the recreation section of this week.

- Be healthy and resilient. Exercise, Yoga and a healthy lifestyle can all increase your resilience to deal with stress.

**Defeat Stress with Optimism:**

Every day, from the moment you wake up until the moment you fall asleep, you have a choice: you can let your mood dictate your day or you can let your day dictate your mood. When you get out of bed, decide that you're going to have a great day! Choose to be happy and don't let life's little problems get you down. Your attitude affects the way you see the world, and if you decide to be in a good mood no matter what, you'll find that life looks a whole lot brighter. Life will never be perfect, so just accept the fact that some rain clouds will come your way every once in a while, and do your best not to let a few rain drops dampen your life and spirit. Have you noticed that the funniest shows on television are the ones where everything seems to go wrong? The next time you find yourself having one of those horrible, not so good days; remind yourself not to take life so seriously. Laugh at yourself when you make a mistake. Laugh and choose to enjoy life. Try not to stress over every little detail or every pound gained. Do your best and then let laughter fill your life. Laugh at what life throws at you, even if it's a curve ball! Have you heard the saying "you'll look back at this one day and laugh?" Choose to laugh about it now! You will feel much better as a result and put less pressure and stress on yourself.

*Being optimistic and choosing to laugh and enjoy life will help you to stress less over things and improve your quality of life.*

Attitude is everything, so decide not to stress as much about your weight. De-stress your life and change your reality. Decide and convince and train yourself that you are a beautiful and magnificent gift. You have great characteristics that you can dwell on. Chances are your body is not as bad as you think it is. Show off the body part that you least like and send it love and affection. Forgive yourself for not being perfect. This connected feeling will resonate and help you connect with your being. Take a mental note of your expectations. Remember, high expectations and comparisons make you sad and add undo pressure in your life. Evaluate what you are expecting of yourself and give yourself credit with your progressions. This is the body given to you in this lifetime, accept it and make it striking. Treasure yourself, your health and reflect constantly on who you are inside. Hold your head up high, and notice the wonderful exquisiteness that lies inside you radiate out; this will speak volumes more than your physical body ever could. An astonishingly perfect body (whatever that might be), is not attractive with an unpleasant soul and pessimistic attitude. Keep upbeat from the inside-out and everything will catch on luminously. Don't be so hard on yourself. By doing so, you create undue stress - stress that releases fat storing hormones, creates poor digestion, eats up your energy, causes excessive eating and sluggish bodily functions. Remove the pressure and focus on self-love.

## Ten ways to reduce stress in your life: Summary

- Add more fun to your life - do things you enjoy and enjoy what you do.

- Get enough sleep and rest - your body must recharge and discharge tensions.

- Express your feelings - unexpressed emotions are the seeds of stress, pain and illness.

- Exercise regularly as it's a great way to relieve tension, increase energy and improve your mood. Find an activity you like and do it often.

- Love more - learn to use things and to love people, instead of the other way around.

- Eliminate self-pity - you may get sympathy for a while, but soon others will want to avoid you.

- Develop meaningful relationships - it is important to have good friends in whom you can confide and find support. It is also important to be a true friend.

- Alter behaviors and attitudes - when ideas or views are not serving you well, change them. Learn how to respond to situations rather than react. Learn to compromise.

- Learn relaxation techniques - meditation, yoga, tai chi and experience inner peace.

- Reconnect with your inner self (your soul). Practice yoga for a deeper relaxation and self-realization.

*The time is now...*

**It's time for self-coaching and inner reflection:**

Take time to answer and work through these questions in your journal to help keep you focused and on a clear path towards your goals. By taking action you will bring your goals into your life. These self-coaching questions will help clarify what you need to have accomplished this week.

### Self-Coaching Questions

- What needs to happen each day this week?
- What are my priorities this week?
- How will these action steps help me get closer to my goals?
- In the next week my complete focus will be on?
- My direction is clear to me because...?
- I am willing to commit to...?
- What might success look like to me for this week?
- What resonated and stood out to me from the program and what impact will it have on me this week?
- I deserve this because...?
- I am thrilled with myself because...?
- Why is it important for me to take action and follow my goals this week?

# — NOTES —

*"Yoga is the practice of quieting the mind."*

— *Patanjali*

# — WEEK SIX —

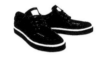

## Recreation Management

Yoga and meditation are fantastic for stress management,
optimism and can help you on your Mission!
How yoga helps reduce anxiety, reduce pessimism
and manages stress.

### What is Yoga?

It seems like a hot new trend, but yoga actually began more than 3000 years ago. The word yoga is Sanskrit (one of the ancient languages of the East). It means to "yoke", or unite or bring together the mind, body and spirit. Although yoga includes physical exercise, it is also a lifestyle practice for which exercise is just one component. Training your mind, body, and breath, as well as connecting with your spirituality, are the main goals in a yoga lifestyle. The physical part of the yoga lifestyle is called Hatha yoga. Hatha yoga focuses on asana, or poses. A person who practices yoga goes through a series of specific poses while controlling his or her breathing. Although there are many different types of yoga, including but not limited to, Ashtanga yoga, Bikram yoga, Gentle yoga, Kundalini yoga, Iyengar yoga, Restorative yoga and Vinyasa/power yoga, they all provide a plethora of health and spiritual benefits. Physically speaking, yoga provides improved flexibility, strength, balance, and stamina. Spiritually speaking, yoga reduces anxiety and stress, improves mental clarity, and even aids in an improved quality of sleep.

## What is Meditation?

Meditation is a method for quieting the mind and replacing business with peace and calm. When our mind is peaceful we are free from worries and mental discomfort, and we experience true happiness. If we train our mind to become peaceful, we will be stress-free most of the time, even in the most adverse conditions. But if our mind is not peaceful, even if we have the most pleasant external conditions we will not be happy. It is therefore important to train our mind through meditation. Meditation is a technique for working with the mind. If you think of the mind as a tool then the first step in putting it to use should be to examine it; reflect on how it works and its possible uses, then put it to work as efficiently and effectively as you can. Meditation is a natural way of getting to know the mind so that we can investigate and understand how it works and then improve it through training. It takes a lot of practice to train the mind. Just as doing weights and jogging make the body fit, practicing meditation makes the mind fit. Looking at the mind in a meditative state leads to understanding, and this leads to freedom from stress and pressure. Meditation is like resting. When you work your body hard you need to take a break. The mind is not any different. All day long your processing information and your mind needs a break. Meditation allows us to relax around stress, problems and issues. It provides opportunity to change the attitude and find peace. In yoga practice, a good portion of the class is devoted to meditation and calming the mind.

### Yoga, meditation and how it can help with stress management:

Everyone suffers from mild anxiety and stress from time to time, but chronic anxiety and stress take a tremendous toll on the body, draining energy resources and keeping the body in a constant state of stress. The effects of anxiety are magnified when the body is not exercised: tension in the muscles builds, breathing remains constricted most of the time, and the mind has no rest from the whirling thoughts and feelings that feed the tension. Yoga helps you to access an inner strength that allows you to face the overwhelming challenges, fears, or frustrations of everyday life. Coping skills built in yoga and meditation practices greatly help in dealing with stress and tension. A few yoga exercises practiced daily help to regulate the breath, connect you to your inner calm, and relax the body by gently releasing tension from the large muscle groups, flushing all parts of the body and brain with fresh blood, nutrients and oxygen - all the while increasing your feelings of well-being. The complete breath taught in yoga practice is a must for anyone who often feels "stressed-out." Once learned, the complete breath can be used anywhere, anytime, to reduce the severity of anxiety and tension, to calm the mind or to cope with a difficult situation. This daily practice of yoga and meditation is essential and can make a profound difference. Whenever you feel overwhelmed, meditation and/or yoga can be your option to get you in touch with your inner resources and enhance greater awareness, leading you to a peaceful place.

### How yoga can help with increased levels of optimism:

A positive mental attitude is vital to successful weight management. But, as anyone who's ever tried to shed a few pounds knows that losing weight is not easy and keeping up the motivation is even harder. Yoga and meditation can help as it tones and trains both the mind and body. As mentioned above, yoga is known for increasing feelings of well-being and strengthening positive mental attitude. Being optimistic can lead you to feel better about yourself and the accomplishments you have made and will continue to make. Choose to be happy about your reality right now and you will be amazed how everything will work for you in the future. When you are optimistic you tend to stress less and notice the blessings all around. Decide to be the person that notices the roses instead of the thorns on rose bushes. In yoga practice, there is a Sanskrit word 'Mudita'; this word reflects the meaning of noticing the rainbows in everything, it means looking for what is great even in the things that might not seem good. Appreciate what is, and let everything else fall away. When we strive for Mudita, this optimistic view, it is amazing how the typical stress that might be present melts away. Pressure is removed when we see the world through rose coloured glasses; yoga helps us see the world in this way.

## How yoga can help on your Mission:

Yoga is renowned for its physical benefits, which include increased flexibility, greater muscle tone and greater balance. Yoga can help you strengthen your muscles, raise your metabolism and contribute to weight-loss. By improving your flexibility and balance while practicing yoga, you will be better equipped and less likely to incur an injury while performing any aerobic or high-impact exercises. Yoga can help relieve stress and tension by stretching muscles, can improve range of motion in the joints and can correct postural imbalances that occur due to weight gain. In addition, yoga can help increase your energy levels, making it easier for you to start and finish your workouts. Because yoga helps put you in touch with your body, it can help you learn to make better dietary decisions by helping you realize which foods strengthen your body and which weaken it. Some weight-loss experts believe that yoga helps regulate your endocrine system to control sleep, appetite and mood. Yoga can also help improve digestion, to eliminate constipation, water retention as well as bloating, all of which may be contributing to your higher weight.

If you're trying to lose weight, chances are good that a negative mental attitude is your biggest obstacle. It's hard to change longtime habits, and many who are struggling to lose weight engage in negative self-talk when they fail to meet their weight-loss goals. Yoga teaches self-acceptance, and can help you learn to love your body as it really is, rather than as you'd like it to be. While this might seem counterproductive to a weight-loss regimen, self-acceptance is key to maintaining a positive mental attitude while you're losing weight. After all, everyone's body type and ideal healthy weight is different. Self-acceptance can help you reach the goal weight that's right for you, and steer you clear of the dangers on the road to weight-loss, such as eating disorders. Many who do yoga say that it helps them feel more in control of their own lives and habits. Maintaining a positive mental attitude about weight-loss can be difficult if you feel like a slave to your own weight. Yoga can help you understand that you can control your weight, rather than letting your weight control you.

### Getting started with yoga and meditation:

Many gyms, community centers, and yoga studios offer yoga classes. Your community may also have specialized yoga studios. Some yoga instructors offer private or semi-private classes for students as well. Before taking a class, check whether the instructor is registered with the Yoga Alliance, a certification that requires at least 200 hours of training in yoga techniques and teaching. You many also want to do a drop-in class before you commit to signing up for a whole session. Many teachers are strong, safe and educated but some are not. If you sit in on some classes and try a few different types of classes, you will eventually find an instructor that has a style right for you and allows you to feel safe and comfortable. If group classes aren't your style, you could also try using a yoga DVD. Websites, DVDs, and books can't compare to learning yoga poses from a teacher, but they can help you find out more and get you started. They can especially be helpful if you have already taken many yoga classes and want to practice at home.

Dress comfortably for your first yoga session in clothing that allows you to move your body fully. Stretchy shorts or pants and a t-shirt or tank top are best. Yoga is practiced barefoot, so you don't have to worry about special shoes. If you are doing your yoga workout on a carpeted floor, you don't really need equipment, although it is advisable to use a yoga mat or "sticky" mat. This special type of mat provides moderate cushioning and grip while you are in the poses. You can buy yoga mats in sporting goods stores or often at the studio class location. Before you begin any type of exercise program, it's a good idea to talk to your doctor, especially if you have a health problem. Be sure to let your instructor know about any special needs you might have before your class starts. A good instructor will be able to provide modified poses for the students who are just beginning or have special needs.

*"The life of inner peace, being harmonious and without stress is the easiest type of existence."*

— Norman Vincent Peale

# — WEEK SIX —

## Nutrition Management

Get diet revenge and combat stress with nutrition. Understanding the link between stress and weight management.

### What stress does to our physiology?

Stress is present in daily life. Some would say it is unavoidable. It can cause many different kinds of health issues as well as affect your weight. But what exactly is the relationship between stress and weight gain? Stress can be defined as any forces from the outside world that affects you. While stress can help you learn and grow, more often it can cause you anxiety and frustration. Stressors are specifically defined by each individual and what may cause stress for you may be taken in stride by others. When you are under stress, many physiological responses can cause weight gain. Have you noticed that each time you stress yourself about losing weight, you can rarely achieve weight loss and you actually end up gaining more weight? Why is this so common? Understanding what happens when you are under stress will explain the seemingly illogical weight gain. Stress causes an actual physical response in your body. When you are under stress, you secrete stress hormones that cause the body to react to the stressful situation. When a threat is perceived, real or imagined, the body has an automatic defense mechanism. This is often called the "fight or flight" response. It is your body's way of protecting you. When this happens, adrenalin and cortisol are released in your bloodstream. Other hormones also released include epinephrine and nor-epinephrine, all these hormones are filtered by the liver. Your breathing becomes rapid. Blood is redirected away from your digestive track and sent to your muscles and limbs. Your impulses quicken, and your pupils dilate. All of these physical reactions are the primitive way your body prepares to meet the perceived threat with which it is faced. Stress and nutrition have a huge connection. Stress can be a problem in itself, of course. But stress can sometimes lead to unhealthy lifestyle patterns which may lead to more stress! You can control your stress effectively with food choices.

### How stress cause weight gain:

There is no doubt we face stress every day, whether our stress comes from work overload, deadlines, traffic, our kids, our spouse, bills or any other stressors that come with a modern lifestyle. We can also put stress on ourselves to be too slim and to lose weight. Mental stress is another major contributor to all the forms of stress in our life, as we've learned in the previous section. These chronic stressors that many of us face each day are unfortunately more trouble than they're worth! Continued stress on the body results in a chronically activated stress response (excess cortisol), and this long-term physiological change to our bodies takes its toll on our health. Clinical studies from Yale University, University of Miami, University of California, University of Connecticut and The University of Chicago, and many other studies around the world, have shown that lowering stress and reducing cortisol to normal levels can reduce body fat levels and control appetite.

**The liver connection in relation to stress:** The liver plays an important role in regulating body weight by playing a role in blood sugar regulation, thyroid regulation and fat metabolism. If stress hormones burden the liver, the liver cannot do its other jobs efficiently, resulting in weight gain and a body that has other poor bodily processes.

**The emotional connection in relation to stress:** Emotional eating and stress from emotional baggage can also contribute to weight struggles. Putting undue emotional pressure on yourself to lose weight increases anxiety and thus increases the stress response which burdens the natural bodily processes. As you know, eating more calories than you burn off causes weight gain. The goal is to find a balance between healthy eating and exercise. Many people have emotional triggers when it comes to unhealthy eating. Bad news can send you to the drive-thru or to the cookie jar. Emotional pressure can also lead to the absence of listening to your inner voice and natural cravings. Applying a positive attitude to counteract the emotional burden will help decrease the strain associated with emotional pressure. For a short time, the enjoyment or positive feeling of eating those chocolate bars, greasy fries, and chips helps you to feel better. This feeling subsides, however, when you realize that you have consumed all of those unwanted calories. That short term comfort turns into discomfort and further upset and this often leads to a vicious cycle. Depression and stress from overeating typically leads to more overeating in an effort to feel good. In this way, stress and/or unhappiness can directly relate to gaining unwanted pounds.

**The blood sugar connection in relation to stress:** Many studies have linked stress with eating behaviour and studies show that not only does stress affect the way we eat, but that the way we eat affects our ability to handle stressful situations. It works in this way: When we don't eat enough food, or don't eat healthy whole food choices, we experience blood sugar level fluctuations. Fluctuations in blood sugar often lead to mood swings, fatigue, poor concentration, as well as other negative reactions. When you have hypoglycemia (low blood sugar), for example, your body does not function as well as it should, you cannot interpret your situation in the same way if your blood sugar levels were properly regulated. For example, how I deal with traffic with low blood sugar levels is very different than when I have just eaten. If I have regulated blood sugar levels my outlook, attention and ability to handle the situation is better. Additionally, stress makes the body crave foods that are high in fats and sugar, which in time will inflict a greater stress on the body and affect blood sugar levels. I used to say to my kids, when their dad got home and he would be grumpy because his blood sugar levels were low, "leave Daddy alone until he gets some food into his belly." There is a direct link to ability to handling stress and blood sugar levels.

**The cortisol connection in relation to stress:** Cortisol is a hormone that is secreted by the adrenal gland. It is involved in many of our body's important functions including regulating blood pressure, glucose metabolism, regulation of insulin release to control blood sugar levels, as well as inflammatory responses. Cortisol is dubbed the "stress hormone" because it is released at high levels when the body is under "stress". The affects of long-term production of cortisol due to chronic stress, for example, have been well documented:

### Here is a list of the physiological and health impacts:

- Impaired cognitive performance
- Suppressed thyroid function
- Blood sugar imbalances such as hyperglycemia
- Decreased bone density
- Decrease in muscle tissue
- Higher blood pressure
- Lowered immunity and inflammatory responses in the body, slowed wound healing, and other health consequences
- Increased abdominal fat, which is associated with a greater amount of health problems than fat deposited in other areas of the body. Some of the health problems associated with increased stomach fat are: heart attacks, strokes, the development of metabolic syndrome, higher levels of "bad" cholesterol (LDL) and lower levels of "good" cholesterol (HDL), which can lead to other health problems.

Stress leads to weight gain primarily because of cortisol being over-secreted. When you are under chronic stress, the amount of cortisol circulating in your body stays elevated, and this prolonged dose of cortisol signals your brain to hold on to your energy stores, a.k.a. fat cells, as the body is tricked into thinking it's under imminent threat. Cortisol also acts as a potent signal to the brain to increase appetite and increase cravings for food especially for carbohydrates and fats. In the modern world, however, we aren't in a life and death situation (hopefully anyway!), and instead, the prolonged elevation of cortisol is unnecessary for our survival. We don't need this huge amount of storage or stock up of energy stores. Further to this, under chronic stress, cortisol slows the body's metabolic rate by blocking the effects of many of your most important metabolic hormones, including insulin (so blood sugar levels suffer and carbohydrate cravings follow), serotonin (so we feel fatigued and depressed), growth hormones (so we lose muscle and gain fat), and the sex hormones testosterone and estrogen (so our sex drive falls). Your body increases glucose levels from the stored glycogen in the liver every time you activate your stress response. This excess sugar combines with insulin and is stored as fat.

Eating to manage stress will work in a similar way. Stress causes stored glycogen to dump in the blood (so it is like eating a chocolate bar) in order to deal with the stress, the blood sugar levels rise and fall, only to encourage the body to eat more to support future stress. The discouraging truth is that stress can make you gain weight and sabotage your efforts to lose weight. Studies have shown that cortisol is elevated when you diet as well. The stress-induced elevations of cortisol levels can strongly influence eating behavior, emotional outlook and body weight. Your body thinks it needs more energy to deal with the stress you are under and encourages hunger.

Controlling stress and cortisol levels is clearly critical to achieving your overall goals of shedding extra body weight. The key is to find what your sources of stress may be. Perhaps it is unrealistic deadlines, a busy schedule, lack of sleep, or family issues? The most important thing to remember is that stress is something that is external; it is how you interpret the event that makes it stressful. Thankfully there are many ways to reduce stress and have a positive impact on your life.

**Combat stress with nutrition:**

Your life is already stressful without having to worry about what goes into your mouth. However, what you eat and how you eat it can contribute to your ability to cope with the stress in your life. Eating the wrong things or eating at the wrong time can add to your stress level. Alternatively the better you eat, the more equipped you are to handle the stressful situation. Learning how to cope with stress and deal with it in a healthy way is far more productive than allowing the stress to negatively impact your body and dealing with the ensuing consequences. You can do without the negative health effects stress has on you! Keeping your blood sugar levels regulated will help you deal with stress favourably and keep you calm.

**Choosing low-stress foods-** The following are some guidelines to help you choose foods to lower your stress levels as well as help your body cope with the stress in your life.

**Include some complex carbohydrates in every meal-** Complex carbohydrates such as rice pasta, ancient grain cereals, oatmeal, potatoes, and brown rice can enhance your performance when under stress. Foods rich in carbohydrates can increase levels of serotonin in the body, making you feel better. Avoid refined flours, wheat products, and too many carbohydrates.

**Reduce your intake of simple carbohydrates-** Sweetened, sugary foods, like soda, candy, and refined sugar should be avoided whenever possible. Simple carbohydrates will make you feel good in the short-term but bad in the long-term. When blood sugar levels drop, your ability to deal with stress drops too. Your brain and thought processes are hindered when blood sugar levels drop off.

**Eat adequate amounts of protein-** This means eating more fish, chicken, eggs, tofu and other sources of lean protein. Foods high in protein enhance mental functioning and supply essential amino acids that can help repair damage to your body's cells. Protein also helps regulate blood sugar levels by regulating the rate of carbohydrate absorption.

**Eat your vegetables-** Broccoli, peppers, carrots, squash and dark green leafy veggies, whether cooked or raw (avoid overcooking), provide your body with the vitamins and nutrients it needs to resist the negative effects of stress and calm your nervous system. Get plenty of potassium. Skim milk, whole grains (rice, spelt, bulgur, etc.), nuts and seeds all can provide your body with potassium, a mineral that can help your muscles relax. Bananas and pumpkin seeds are also a good source of potassium and also help regulate blood pressure and support the heart.

**Increase vitamin B rich foods-** B vitamins are often referred to as the "stress vitamins". B vitamins may help you to stay calm and deal with stress in a positive manner. They are also essential for the functioning of the heart, the muscles and the nervous system. Vitamins B3 and B6 are especially important because they help supply fuel to cells, which are then able to burn energy and function optimally. When cells are functioning well you are better able to deal with stress and make rational evaluations of events. Vitamin B6 together with zinc is necessary for the production of pancreatic enzymes which help you digest food. If your digestion is good, your body will be more likely to use your food efficiently, instead of storing food as fat. These vitamins also provide you with energy and allow for carbohydrate, fat and protein metabolism. B vitamins are important for the release of energy. They are also needed for the maintenance of healthy skin, nerves, and the gastrointestinal tract. In terms of weight-loss, B vitamins provide you with energy to burn more calories as they are needed for the proper function of the thyroid gland and metabolism. They also play a part in glucose tolerance factor (GTF) which is released every time blood sugar levels rise. When you can tolerate glucose efficiently, you have more consistent blood sugar levels. This will help you deal better with stress and not store as much fat in response to fluctuating blood sugar levels. Vitamin B5 is involved in energy production and helps to control fat metabolism. B-rich foods include: whole grain products, rice, oatmeal, legumes, eggs, cheese, peas, green leafy vegetables, whole grain cereals, molasses, avocados, bananas and cabbage. A good quality, B-complex vitamin is highly recommended – it's important to take as a group in addition to eating B rich foods.

**Stress-busting snacking-** Feeling anxious, nervous, stressed out? Need a quick food fix? Snacking, when done right, is an art. Anyone can grab a donut or chips and a pop. The real skill is coming up with a snack that doesn't add to your stress level and helps you reduce the stress you already have. Snacking is important to keep your blood sugar levels up so you can deal with stress and day to day living more effectively. Avoid highly sugared treats. They will give you a boost in the short-term but let you down in the long-term when your blood sugar levels drop too drastically. Stick with snacks that have high-energy proteins and are high in complex carbohydrates, fiber and nutrients. They will give you a longer lasting, sustained pick-me-up. Snack at regular intervals between meals as this will help to regulate blood sugar levels and boost metabolism; both essential for weight and stress management. Quick bites and snacks can boost your mood and help alleviate some of your stress.

### Here are some snack suggestions:

- Fruit
- Trail mix
- Raw or lightly roasted unsalted nuts
- Dates, raisins, apricots, figs, and other dried fruit (look for 'unsulphured')
- Fruit leathers
- Apple sauce (without added sugar)
- Raw vegetables with optional dip (use home-made dips or hummus with natural ingredients)
- Celery stuffed with nut butter
- Sandwiches on rye or whole grain breads
- Soup (home-made if possible - avoid canned soups)
- Blender drinks (smoothies)
- Muffins, cookies, loaves (home-made or made with natural sweeteners like honey and no preservatives)
- Yogurt (avoid ones with added sugar - particularly artificial sugar such as sucralose)

- Popcorn (organic, or no-salt options)
- Rice crackers or ancient grain crackers with non-processed cheeses (choose low-sodium options)
- Rice cakes with nut butter or apple sauce and a sprinkle of cinnamon
- Rye crisps with spreads (hummus is great)
- Oatmeal (home-made, or choose the plain instant without added preservatives and chemicals)
- Organic corn chips with salsa

**Please take a mental note:** Too much of a good thing is no longer a good thing either. Snacking can cause extra calories to enter your body. The secret is to eat more frequently but not more quantity.

### Avoid using food as therapy for stress:

Stress can cause you to use food as a form of therapy or relaxation. Learn what makes you eat besides hunger. We consume foods for nourishment, but we also consume foods out of insecurities such as loneliness, boredom, procrastination, habit and comfort. It is important to pinpoint what it is that drives you to eat when you're not hungry and don't require food. Once you isolate the issues, it becomes easy to recognize the patterns and begin to change the behavior. Learning to deal with emotions and stress can have a profound effect on weight management. Be aware of emotional eating. It will only help you with stress in the short-run and make you feel guilty and terrible in the long-run. Look to other means for consolation and choose stress effective eating.

*"It's not stress that kills us; it is our reaction to it."*

— *Hans Selye*

Being optimistic and choosing to laugh and enjoy life will help you to stress less over things and improve your quality of life. Stress isn't always bad. In small doses, it can help you perform under pressure and motivate you to do your best at a task. Stress is present in daily life. Some would say it is unavoidable. It can cause many different kinds of health issues as well as affect your weight. You know you can get diet revenge and combat stress with nutrition. Understanding the link between stress and weight management is just the first step in combatting the impact it could have on you. Managing stress is all about taking action and personal responsibility: taking charge of your thoughts, your emotions, your time, your environment, and the way you respond with problems. Stress management is about avoiding unnecessary stress, changing the situation if you can, positively Adapting to the situation, accepting things that you can't change, take on a healthy lifestyle and getting plenty of sleep. Further to that, yoga and meditation are great ways to de-stress and put things into perspective.

# STAY ON TARGET

## MY WEEKLY CHECKLIST

- [x] Choose to be optimistic
- [x] Stress less
- [x] Combat stress with Yoga
- [x] Accept things you can't change
- [x] Manage stress with nutrition
- [x] Find ways to de-stress
- [ ] _____
- [ ] _____
- [ ] _____
- [ ] _____
- [ ] _____
- [ ] _____
- [ ] _____
- [ ] _____
- [ ] _____
- [ ] _____
- [ ] _____

## MY WEIGHT THIS WEEK:

Began at:_____

Finished at:_____

Total weight loss:_____

## MY MEASUREMENTS THIS WEEK:

### BEGAN AT

Shoulders:_____

Chest:_____

Waist:_____

Hips:_____

### FINISHED AT

Shoulders:_____

Chest:_____

Waist:_____

Hips:_____

### DIFFERENCE/TOTAL INCHES LOST:

Shoulders:_____

Chest:_____

Waist:_____

Hips:_____

What really resonated for me this week?

_____
_____
_____
_____
_____
_____
_____
_____
_____
_____
_____

What worked well for me this week?

_____
_____
_____
_____
_____
_____
_____
_____
_____
_____
_____
_____

# WEEK SEVEN

# Psychology Management/Self-Coaching

Its time to step it up a notch with tough love this week!
Excuses and self-pity can deflate you on your Mission,
it's time to take responsibility for your life.

# Recreation Management

Learn how to plan and build workouts and active living
into your life. Learn tricks to optimize your exercise plan
and fit activity into your schedule.

# Nutrition Management

Planning your nutrition for the week will help you on your
Mission. Menu planning and preparation contributes to
healthy eating and natural weight balancing.

*"In the long run, we shape our lives, and we shape ourselves. The process never ends until we die. And the choices we make are ultimately our own responsibility."*

— *Eleanor Roosevelt*

# — WEEK SEVEN —

## Psychology Management/Self- Coaching

It's time to step it up a notch with tough love this week!
Excuses and self-pity can deflate you on your Mission,
it's time to take responsibility for your life.

Welcome to week seven of Mission Slim Possible! This week will allow you to explore how taking personal responsibility for your level of success on your Mission can drive positive change, both in your weight-balancing approach as well as in your life overall.

This week I encourage you to step things up a notch, eliminate or minimize any self-pity or excuses and replace it with full active responsibility for your life and results. You will learn how to plan and build workouts and active living into your life. Planning your nutrition for the week will help you on your Mission.  Menu planning and preparation contribute to healthy eating and natural weight balancing. It's time to step it up a notch with tough love this week! Excuses and self-pity can deflate you on your Mission, it's time to take responsibility and accountability for your life.

*"The only thing feeling sorry for yourself changes about your life, is that it makes it worse." - Guy Finley*

### What are excuses?

What's your exercise excuse? What's your overeating excuse? What's your lack of motivation excuse? What is your health excuse? We all collect a shortlist of the most common excuses for not making our goals or Mission become a reality. I have to say I have heard almost every excuse in the book form clients, friends, students, and my kids. Oh and, yes, I have a fair share of my own excuses. In psychology and logic, rationalization (also known as making excuses) is a defense mechanism we use to make ourselves feel better about not measuring up to where we would like to be. An excuse is an attempt to lessen blame or a desire to defend or justify. An excuse example might be, "it is totally hormonal for me" or " my kids keep me too busy, I can't make it to the gym." An excuse is the attempt to pardon or forgive incompetence. Those who specialize in excuses seldom accomplish what they set out to accomplish. A rationalization is a reason that a person might give to explain why you did something wrong or out of line. This defense mechanism hides or conceals your true motivation by explaining your actions and feelings in a way that is not as threatening or harsh. It is actually a cognitive process of making something seem real, or an excuse or reason for not measuring up, be explained or justified. In other words, "not enough time in a day" excuse for not losing weight, is a rationalization of not meeting your target.

## What is self-pity?

Self-pity, like excuses, is a psychological state of mind, where individuals believe that they are a victim. They think they have done no wrong and the negative situation they find themselves in is a result of outside sources. Self-pity is the emotion of denying oneself of confidence. It is the belief that you are a victim and have no or little control over your current situation. To experience self-pity, is to feel sorry for yourself. Self-pity tends to be stultifying and inactive and goes hand and hand with excuses. Some psychologists believe that depression has its roots in self-pity or in 'poor me' thinking. I believe self-pity is easily one of the most destructive habits that does not serve people positively and hinders positive change. I let myself feel good and sorry for myself, but only for a moment. Then I move out of that self-pity mode as fast as possible and take action towards positive change for myself. Self-pity is not only unattractive; when we have problems, all we see are the problems and that's all we start to talk about. Self-pity takes you into a negative mind-set and sets you up for excuse and external blame mode.

## Why are excuses and self-pity negative on your Mission?

Along your Mission, it is extremely important to take positive action towards your goals you set out for yourself. Consider the biggest thing holding you back from your life goals may be yourself? But often, people fall back onto excuses and self-pity and give up trying to reach their goals. When you are wrapped up in self-pity, you can completely spoil any chance of being able to see new possibilities as they appear. The only thing that grows from self-pity or feeling sorry for oneself is bitter, negative experiences. Feeling sorry for yourself is a slow acting poison. The only thing really standing in your way between you and your goal is lame excuses that you are not good enough or have roadblocks in the way to achieving your goal. By agreeing to live with sad regrets or in self-pity, you only ensure they will still be with you tomorrow. Sorry for sounding harsh, but you get the point that self-pity and feeling sorry for yourself does not work to your advantage. Self-pity gives power to those you blame for your own situation. First, it corrupts, and then it consumes you and chokes you. Do you know people who have excuses, or more likely "reasons" for not being a certain size, weight, fitness level? Think about how painful it is to hear people's excuses and complaining. Do you want to be one of those people, heck no! You're on a MISSION! "Poor me, poor me, poor me" does make us feel better temporarily, and that is important to do. You need some level of soothing when things do go bad. But that's all it does, self-pity needs to be temporary and limited. Self-pity will not do anything towards healing the damage, fixing the problem, or bettering our lives. Any time you place responsibility for a situation or outcome entirely outside of yourself, you also place the ability to remedy or fix the situation entirely outside of yourself. That is very disempowering and destructive on your way towards your target.

Conversely, self-pity brings you down and sets you up for a future of struggle and lack of goal achievement. Self-pity exists as a real emotion. All real emotions do have both sides, a positive and a negative side. The small positive side of pity and excuses comes with its powers of calming or numbing the pain. In fact, I believe self-pity and excuses could be very addictive. It serves people well in the short term and as a basis for survival, but, on the negative side, self-pity and excuses can paralyze your thoughts and feelings, and even your actions. The person swamped with self-pity and excuses really is leading a sad life, filled with problems and struggle. Life is difficult when you're drowning in self-pity. Bad things really do happen. And one of the characteristics of pity is that you always have someone to blame, even if it's blaming yourself. These individuals usually look outside of themselves for the source of their problems and struggle. Remember, you create your reality with your thoughts, feelings and attitudes. You attract into your life what you think about most of the time! By definition, a person having self-pity cannot, and will not, accept responsibility for their own life. Someone else must be responsible. Flush any excuses and self-pity down the drain. Choose to look for your success and accomplishments instead of your short-comings.

### How to stop excuses and self-pity?

How often do you find yourself coming up with a myriad of "reasons" why you have not yet accomplished your goals or achieved the level of success you desire? I started noticing at one point in my life, I kept finding myself saying, "There is not enough time in a day." I realized I kept using this reason, limited time, as a excuse for not meeting my targets. Once I started realizing that this was an excuse and self-pity, I adopted a "no excuse" line of thinking and things began to change. I changed my statement, so it would be more productive, to " I make maximum use of my time." It was amazing how I was able to build into my life the time I needed to get back on target. True, I had to start waking up at 6am, but at least I was getting the time I needed to stay true to my Mission. If you want something bad enough you can find the motivation to work towards it, eliminating excuses, reasons and self-pity. I suggest that you first look where you find yourself making excuses in your life. Does it serve you in any way? If not, I suggest you adopt the "no excuse" thinking. Accept that your life will be busy, lacking in time, have challenges, kids, relationships, work, etc., and not let it get you down and off target.

People duck responsibility for reasons ranging from fear of failure or laziness, through to a sense of feeling overwhelmed by unrealistic targets or tough situations. Whatever the reason, if people don't take responsibility, they'll fail to grow and learn as an individual. All of this makes it very important to address typical places we use excuses and self-pity. Some warning signs you are using this destructive tool are: blaming others for mistakes or failures, missing goals, avoiding challenging tasks or projects, regularly complaining about your current situation, avoiding taking initiative, and being dependent on others, making excuses regularly. Sometimes, people feel as if they have no control over their lives and situation. To them, it doesn't matter what they do or how hard they work, nothing makes much difference in their eyes. It is a matter to shifting this thinking to that of taking responsibility and control of your life that allows you to feel empowered.

You are a strong and worthy person! Take back your power and take notice when you go into "poor me" excuse or self-pity mode. Don't let "poor me" be how you take care of yourself when you've felt wronged or didn't meet your target. Lick your wounds for a few moments, or longer if you need, but set a time limit on how long you'll indulge in this mode and then take charge and be proactive. Drop the self-pity, close that door and state to yourself, "I'm not doing excuses anymore!" Figure out how you contributed to the unhappy, unpleasant situation in which you find yourself, or how you allowed it to come about in the first place, and then take responsibility and do what it takes to either transform the present situation or make sure things turn out differently moving forward.

### How to take responsibility for your life:

As a part of a successful weight-balancing program, you need to honor and recognize your success and move away from self-pity and excuses. Step it up a notch, and give recognition to the need of taking personal responsibility. You need to honor and celebrate the achievements you have made and the successful strides you have achieved. In fact, recognition and motivation are an integral part of reaching your goals. Acknowledgement and encouragement impact the success of all participants in any weight management program, often catapulting you to the next level of success. This approach will move you away from self-pity and feeling sorry for yourself to a place of action.

It is time to take responsibility for your life, by acknowledging who you are and where you are because of your actions and behavior up until this point. If you want to have a life makeover and reach your target, you need to take ownership for your current situation and the role you play moving forward. Personal responsibility means you behave your way towards your success. Create what you want in your life now, so it shows up in the future as well. You choose your behaviour and you choose the consequences of that behaviour. You need to be held accountable for your life. You have to accept that you have created the life and reality you live in. Throw away your crutches of blame, excuses and self pity, replace it with learning how to take accountability for your actions. Learning how to take accountability for your life, takes a lot of work, but when you are personally accountable, you take ownership that you're involved in and therefore, can influence your life. In other words, only you can decide to build into your life, what you need to have present, to get the results you desire. Your Mission is entirely up to you! The word "accountable" itself means responsible, or taking responsibility for one's actions. So when we're talking about people and being on your Mission, the question becomes, how will you make sure your accounting for your actions? In other words, how will you take responsibility for your behaviour after the fact? And how can you create an action plan of responsibility before you behave inappropriately according to your target.

*"A sign of wisdom and maturity is when you come to terms with the realization that your decisions cause your rewards and consequences. You are responsible for your life, and your ultimate success depends on the choices you make." - Denis Waitley, author and coach*

Successful people take personal responsibility for their lives. They act in ways that produce more of what they want and less of what they don't want. Action might begin with some self-reflection that involves asking yourself; how did I contribute to that? What excuses have I used in the past? What were my beliefs on this issue? What do I need to do differently? What is working? What isn't working? What did I do or not do to create this reality? Successful people respond mindfully to situations and take responsibility for actions. The quality of your life and level of success is up to you. It is your responsibility. No magic pills, fad diet, secret workout or anything alike will help you lose weight, nor will any excuse or self pity justify weight gain, only you are responsible for your level of success.

When you are more receptive to your success and goal accomplishments, it shrinks the need for excuses and self-pity. Remember, self-pity gets attention in the short term but people will avoid you in the long term. People can see through self-pity as excuses. So, choose to take full responsibility for your reality and take action to change what you desire. Notice your success and focus on what needs to happen to get you closer to your goals. You create the life you live! You choose the size of your clothes. You choose the way your body will look.

*"If it's never our fault, we can't take responsibility for it. If we can't take responsibility for it, we'll always be its victim." - Richard Bach*

### How to step your Mission up a notch:

It is time to step your Mission up a notch. This expression means move your self up a level. One of my mentors, Anthony Robbins often says something along the lines of. "why be great when you can be outstanding." This to me, is so super motivating. Why not become the person you want to be? Why not be the best version of yourself? It is possible to be happy right now while striving to be the best version of yourself. Become aware and appreciate all the things you already are doing that bring out your best and get you closer to your target. Love your day and plan your days to support your target. Try to avoid saying "should have" and replace with, "I am going to..." My dad used to say to me while growing up, "Nothing worth doing in life is ever easy." He demonstrated through hard work and dedication, you will be successful. Take on the challenge, embark on the road to self motivated success. It will make you happy in the long run. You pay a huge price when you engage in distraction off your target. That is why engaging yourself into full responsibility and accountability for your actions, is important. I encourage you to wear clothes that fit and flatter your body and make you feel good. Step up your game. Step up your standards. It is time to take yourself to the next level.

### Here are some positive affirmations to help you take responsibility and accountability for your life while on your Mission.

Try these positive affirmations; they'll help you break out of your self-pity trap and feel good about yourself. (Taken from www.freeaffirmations.org) I highly recommend this website to help you with affirmations.

### Present-tense affirmations:

- I am strong.
- I am confident.
- I love myself for who I am.
- I am understood.
- I am appreciated.
- I stand up for myself and my beliefs.
- I stand by my opinions.
- I take responsibility for my actions.
- I am grateful for myself.
- I focus on the positive things in my life.

### Future-tense affirmations

- I will stop wallowing in self-pity.
- I will develop realistic goals for myself.
- I am becoming more self-confident.
- My self-esteem is growing.
- I will focus on doing things for others.
- I will stop giving up.
- I will pursue my dreams.
- I will be proud of myself for who I am.
- I will stop thinking about myself.
- I will buckle down on defeating my self-pity.

### Neutral affirmations

- I know that I am good enough.
- I have full confidence in myself.
- Others see me as strong and well-opinionated.
- I always give to others.
- I am caring and considerate.
- I simply keep the focus off of myself.
- I ignore vanity.
- I avoid feeling sorry for myself.
- I am strong enough to rise above self-pity.
- I am aware of myself and my thoughts.

**It's time for self-coaching and inner reflection:**

Take time to answer and work through these questions in your journal to help keep you focused and on a clear path towards your goals. By taking action you will bring your goals into your life. These self-coaching questions will help clarify what you need to have accomplished this week.

### Self-Coaching Questions

- What needs to happen each day this week?
- What are my priorities this week?
- How will these action steps help me get closer to my goals?
- In the next week my complete focus will be on?
- My direction is clear to me because...?
- I am willing to commit to...?
- What might success look like to me for this week?
- What resonated and stood out to me from the program and what impact will it have on me this week?
- I deserve this because...?
- I am thrilled with myself because…?
- Why is it important for me to take action and follow my goals this week?

# — NOTES —

*"A healthy body is a guest chamber for the soul; a sick body is a prison."*

— *Francis Bacon*

# — WEEK SEVEN —

## Recreation Management

Learn how to plan and build workouts and active living into your life. Learn tricks to optimize your exercise plan and fit activity into your schedule.

**The benefits of being active:**

Being active should be an important part of your every day routine. It helps you burn up excess energy (calories) and helps prevent excess weight gain. Moreover, exercise helps strengthen your bones and muscles, keeps your body healthy, and makes you feel good too. Being active doesn't always mean having to do exercise like going to the gym or getting out on a football field, it's much more than that. Everyday activity such as walking, dancing, gardening, cycling to work, or helping around the house, all count! When you know the benefits of being active, it is that much easier to incorporate activity into your life. Being active will help you feel much fitter and healthier. People who are "always on the go" use and burn more energy and are less likely to become overweight. Increasing activity burns more calories and increases muscle mass, which helps you to lose excess weight. Being active causes your brain to release endorphins and other feel-good hormones that help you feel less stressed and better about yourself. These chemicals give you a natural buzz and feeling of wellbeing. This can help you cope with stressful times in your life. By being active you'll help to keep yourself healthy by strengthening your bones and muscles and keeping your heart and lungs healthy. Being active can help improve your confidence levels and can help you feel better about yourself. Being out and about active and trying new activities means there will be more opportunities for you to meet new people and make new friends.

**How to build activity into your life:**

Finding the time and interest to build physical activity into your daily life could sometimes be difficult. My sister always amazes me. She is one of, if not, the busiest people that I know. She works full time, has two daughters that are in every sport and are competitive gymnasts, she always has something on the go and in addition to all this, races mountain biking. Needless to say, if she can fit training into her hectic, crazy busy life, I think you can. She never ceases to amaze me with her level of motivation and commitment to her fitness. She lives the saying, "Where there is a will, there is a way." We can all come up with lots of excuses to avoid exercise. Let's take the time to look at some of the common barriers people raise, and offer some tips on how to move past them. Is life conspiring to keep you away from the gym and not active this week? Fear not! The following tips will help keep you strong, slender and on your Mission towards your target.

### Some common excuses:

- "I don't have enough time"
- "Exercise is boring"
- "I'm too tired"
- "I don't feel good"
- "I don't feel like it"
- "I don't know how to be active"
- "It's too hot, too cold, it's raining…"

## Some solutions to these common excuses:

- Keep a diary of your daily activities for a week.
- Use a diary to assess how much spare time you actually have – you may have more time than you thought.
- Take a brisk 15-minute walk at lunchtime.
- Exercise with a friend, join a local walking group, or take up a sport.
- Change the way you think about physical activity. Don't think that exercise must be painful or a burden in order to be 'good' for you.
- Mix it up. Plan to participate in a range of physical activities.
- Pick something that really interests you. Join a tennis league for example.
- Find out about opportunities for joining local groups.
- Choose an activity that feels comfortable.
- Try to be active on most days and you'll soon start to feel more energetic and less tired.

- If finding a spare 30 minutes each day to exercise is challenging for you, try to break up your exercise time into two 15-minute bursts, or even into three 10-minute bursts. You'll still benefit from the fitness!

- Don't push yourself too hard. Gradually increase the time and intensity as your fitness improves.

- Choose weather-specific activities such as skiing or snow-play in winter or swimming and outdoor walking in summer.

- Rearrange your schedule to fit fitness into your life.

- Identify your barriers to physical activity and try to create options around those barriers.

- Choose solitary workouts like an exercise video if you feel uncomfortable exercising with other people.

- Make sure your goals are reasonable.

- Plan ahead for periods and time of physical activity. Make appointments in your agenda with yourself. Book it like you would a meeting or appointment.

- Find yourself an exercise buddy to meet regularly. You are more likely to commit to regular physical activity if you have someone else relying on you to show up.

- The best physical activity you can choose is the one you enjoy because that is the one that you will be able to maintain.

- Find the physical activities that appeal to you the most and don't be afraid to try something new. Exercise doesn't have to be dull.

### Fitting fitness into your life

According to the Mayo Clinic, time spent at home doesn't have to be "couch potato" time. You can also make time at work an opportunity for an active life. To make fitness a priority at home or at work, the Mayo Clinic suggests the following:

**Wake up early:** Get up 30 minutes earlier than you normally do and use the extra time to walk on your treadmill or take a brisk walk around the neighborhood.

**Make chores count:** Mop the floor, scrub the bathtub or do other housework at a pace fast enough to get your heart pumping. Outdoor work counts, too. Mowing the lawn with a push mower is a great way to burn calories. Raking and hoeing strengthen your arms and back, and digging works your arms and legs.

**Be active while watching television:** Use hand weights, ride a stationary bike or do a stretching routine during your favorite shows. Get off the couch to change the channel or adjust the volume.

**Involve the whole family:** Take group walks before or after dinner. Play catch. Ride your bikes. It's best to build up to about 30 minutes of continuous activity, but you can exercise in shorter bursts, too.

**Get your dog into the act:** Take daily walks with Fido or Fluffy. If you don't have a dog, borrow one. An enthusiastic dog may give you the motivation you need to lace up your walking shoes.

**Make the most of your commute to work:** Walk or bike to work. If you ride the bus, get off a few blocks early and walk the rest of the way.

**Take the stairs whenever you can:** If you have a meeting on another floor, get off the elevator a few floors early and use the stairs. Better yet, skip the elevator entirely.

**Take fitness breaks at work:** Rather than hanging out in the lounge with coffee or a snack, take a short walk.

**Start a lunchtime walking group at work:** The regular routine and the support of your co-workers may help you stick with the program.

**Put it on the calendar:** Schedule physical activity as you would any other appointment during the day. Don't change your exercise plans for every interruption that comes along.

**Take it on the road:** If you travel for work, plan ahead. Bring your jump-rope or choose a hotel that has fitness facilities. If you're stuck in an airport waiting for a plane, grab your bags and take a walk.

**Get more out of errands:** When you go to the mall or grocery store, park toward the back of the lot and walk the extra distance. If you have a little extra time, walk inside for a lap or two before you start shopping. Keep a pair of walking shoes in your car so that you're ready when you find a few minutes for exercise.

**Plan active outings:** Make a date with a friend to hike in a local park, or take a family trip to the zoo.

**Get social:** Try a dance club, hiking group or golf league. Encouragement from others can help you stay with a new activity.

**Join a team:** Sign up for a softball, soccer or volleyball team through your local parks and recreation department. Making a commitment to a team is a great motivator.

**Join a fitness club:** Sign up for a group exercise class at a nearby fitness club. The cost may be an added incentive to stick with it.

You are well aware that fitness and active living is important for your health and well-being. And you want to get more active for your Mission, but your days are a busy blur of work, household chores, errands, and time with family and friends. Setting aside enough time to sleep, let alone exercise, can be tough. It can be a challenge, but if you take personal responsibility for your Mission, you can build activity into you life. There's no single best way to fit physical activity into your day, only you will be able to create that for yourself. Your lifestyle, job and family responsibilities will point to the most convenient time and place for fitness. Do what works for you, and make daily physical activity and fitness a habit you plan to keep! Use these wonderful tips from the Mayo Clinic to help counteract any excuse. If you come up with a new one, take initiative to come up with solutions to get active for yourself.

*"Productivity is never an accident. It is always the result of a commitment to excellence, intelligent planning, and focused effort."*

— *Paul J. Meyer*

# — WEEK SEVEN —

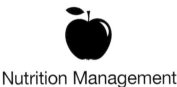

## Nutrition Management

Planning your nutrition for the week will help you on your Mission. Menu planning and preparation contributes to healthy eating and natural weight balancing.

Do you come home from the office tired and wishing you didn't have to think about dinner? Are you home all day with little ones and the last thing you want to do when they go down for a nap is to be busy in the kitchen? Do you open the fridge ready to come up with a good meal only to find you need to run to the grocery store because you're out of an ingredient or two? Do you feel family pressure when it comes to meal time? There is a remedy for all of this. Planning meals is an activity that can bring a number of benefits. You can be cooking for one or an entire family, taking the time to sit down and plan out future meals will not only save you time, effort and money but can help you on your Mission. By planning your meals in advance you can eliminate the last minute rush, poor eating choices, the stress of indecision, and free up more time for your family. Follow your plans and you can achieve your goals. You will eat healthier with thought instead of eating out of starvation and lack of planning.

## The benefits of meal planning:

1. Eat healthier and waste less food- When you know what you're going to eat for dinner that evening, you're less likely to take easy fast food options. Planning your family meals in advance will cut down the amount of pizza or fast food you have delivered to your door. Making a meal from scratch may sound like a hassle but it's a great way to make sure you're eating healthy food. Food you prepare at home tends to be much healthier. When you plan your meals in advance, you will make healthier choices like having chicken breast, as well as some salads and vegetables. Your entire family will benefit from the healthier meals. Most people throw away a lot of food from poor planning. If you only shop and buy what you need for the meals during the week, you will waste less food. Anything that is left over from one meal can be eaten for lunch or snack the next day. When you already have a menu of the foods you are going to prepare for the next couple days, you won't have a chance to eat out or stray from the plan. You will also enjoy variety, which is healthy for the taste buds. Instead of eating the same dish five times a week, you can plan your menu so you are enjoying something new.

2. You'll spend less time in the grocery store- How much time are

you spending running to the grocery store each week? Planning your meals for a week at a time and then putting together a specific grocery list with everything you need, will cut down on your trips to the store to once per week. Not only will you get through your shopping trips much more quickly, you'll make fewer trips. You will also only buy what you need. This alone will save you in time. You shop more efficiently when you have a plan.

3. Save money- By working out your meal in advance, you'll save money in food costs. All that eating out and having food delivered can quickly add up. By preparing more meals at home you will save each week. You will also save on your monthly grocery bill since you will be making a list of everything you need for the week and won't be buying extras that just go to waste. Planning what you'll eat means that you're less likely to fall for impulse buys. I bet you grocery stores don't like when people come in with lists and stick to them. You spend less, and are less likely to impulse buy foods that you don't need. Once you know what ingredients you will be needing, you can also find where to get these ingredients on sale, perhaps and save even more money.

4. Less stress and more quality time- Since meal planning is the advanced planning of meals for the next few days, you don't have to think and can relax around the pre plan. You probably know the routine; it's six o'clock and everyone in the family is starving and you have no idea what to make for dinner, searching the fridge and freezer. Trying to come up with something to cook from what you have in the kitchen when your kids are tired, hungry and ready to eat 'NOW,' isn't one of the most fun family activ-

ities! It can be stressful. You will be much more relaxed around dinner time when you know exactly what you are going to cook ahead of time and you have everything you need to cook in the house. Even still, the meat is already defrosted and ready to go! Stress is minimal when you have a plan and have prepared. Meal time can then be quality time together, free of stress. Dinnertime can be a great time for families share news and experiences of the day. Cook some dinner, set the table and don't forget to turn off the television. You can make dinner time and preparation a daily family tradition again if you like.

**NOTE:** Be flexible with menu planning though. Although there are benefits to meal planning, try to remain flexible. Planning takes a lot of effort and time so you could just plan a few meals. Remember your schedule and plans sometimes change. Modern life can be unpredictable. It's likely something will come up. So be flexible if things don't go as perfectly planned.

### Getting started with menu planning:

Meal planning is a great way to get organized. Give family and personal meal planning a try. I am sure you and your family will see the benefits right away; benefits that go far beyond weight- loss and management. Since you now know all the benefits or menu planning, it is time to get started.

**Start with your main meals -** You can start with just your main bigger meals and eventually roll your planning into every meal. It tends to be the one time of the day where you're at home to eat a proper meal, a non rushed meal. I suggest starting with this main meal first.

**Core or regular meals** - Some dishes you gravitate toward and enjoy eating regularly, these are your core meals or regular meals. These are the meals you can also whip together in a blink of an eye and you feel comfortable preparing. These are good meals to plan on busy nights when following a recipe isn't likely. Build core meals into your busy week.

**Plan your week** - Plan your meals a week in advance. Sit down with cookbooks and write down one or two recipes you would like to try for the week. Know what your week is going to look like. If you know you have a meeting, or company coming, you will have to make special plans around your schedule. Poll your family members for a favorite dish they would like to have and create a meal plan menu chart or simply put it into the family calendar. Put the meals you can prepare with your eyes closed on your busiest evenings. Pick at least one new recipe each week to eliminate boredom and introduce variety. Put the core or regular meals into your week. When healthy options are available it is amazing how easy it is to eat nutritionally dense and healthy foods. Not only will you manage your weight well, the whole family will benefit!

**Create ingredient lists** - Look through the ingredients of each of the recipes you have planned for the week. Take note of what you already have and start creating a list of what you do need. Add these ingredients to the shopping list.

**Make a shopping list** - Keep an ongoing shopping list on your fridge or handy in th kitchen and as you discover things you need you can add them easily to your list. This makes shopping time easier and efficient. Take the sample menu plan for the week and add any ingredients you need to your list. If you are busy and shopping seems like a chore, consider a delivery service. This is more common than you think. Buy only the ingredients on your grocery list, avoid getting distracted. It's also important to shop without your kids and when you are not hungry to avoid buying unnecessary items. The exception to this rule is if something is on sale for a really good price and you want to stock up on the item.

**Remind yourself of the plan** - Hang a piece of paper on the fridge or have it handy in the kitchen or calendar, reminding you of the five to seven meals for the week you have planned.

**Organize your preparation** - Now that you have your recipes and planned meals each day, take some time to read over what is required to prepare the meal and have all the ingredients ready on hand. My favourite part of getting groceries, is coming home and getting every thing washed, chopped and prepared for easy access. Take the time to prep for your meals before you begin - even days ahead ingredients can be prepared to minimize your time in the kitchen. Chop onions and freeze them. See which meats need to be marinated. Chop up your vegetables so they are ready for snacks throughout the week. Start lunches the night before and finish them up in the morning to ease the pressure of the morning rush. Clean all the fruit as soon as you get it home for easy grabbing and to keep longer.

**Keep track of favorite meals (new core meals)** - Record the meals that were a success and plan to do these more often. Make sure you make note of which recipes are keepers. Have a meal-planning section on the calendar. I add meal plans right onto my family calendar, that way I know what we're eating and when. This will help you with meal planning in the future. After a while, all you will have are winning stress-free healthy meals!

## The benefits of being prepared:

Self-improvement is a process whereby we enhance our knowledge in many areas. We do not limit ourselves to any one area of knowledge. Being prepared can reduce fear, anxiety, and losses that accompany not being prepared. Being prepared is essential for self-improvement. Preparation enables us to be ready for future demands and helps us to make great choices and decisions. To prepare is to be ready beforehand for some purpose, situations, use or activity. Athletes do it, sports teams do it, airline pilots do it, professionals do it: Successful people prepare. The hours you spend preparing makes for more positive, more uplifting, more successful life. In terms of nutrition, life throws the unexpected at us every day. From that meeting going overtime, to traffic, to the child who wakes up sick in the middle of the night, we deal with changes to our plans all the time, so it can be particularly difficult at times to manage meals and keep them healthy and nutritious. Being in charge of your life by preparing for those uncontrollable and often unexpected situations will allow you to make the best food choices in any circumstance, such as bringing along prepared and easy to grab snacks or meals with you. Being prepared is an optimistic way to going about life. Being prepared allows you to focus your efforts, plan for success and be great. The next time you find yourself in an unexpected circumstance where it would be easy to grab a burger and fries, give yourself the gift of knowing that you've got what you need, to be able to meet life's emergencies, big and small, with confidence and security. Get prepared!

## Some samples of meal ideas:

The following is just a sample of the many possibilities out there to eat wholesome and nutrient dense foods. Many different things will affect your selection of foods such as nutritional needs, health concerns or allergies, cravings, time of year, which foods are in season, etc., so make choices accordingly. Most importantly, listen to your body and its needs. When you are hungry ask yourself: "What would I love to eat right now?" and you will probably steer towards something in particular. You are learning the tools to eat nutrient dense healthy meals. Selecting two recipes a week is a great way to introduce new foods to the family and yourself and can help create new favorites. Start a folder of all you favorite recipes. Adjust the recipes with your knowledge of whole grains and natural sweeteners and you will have a masterpiece!

## Sample breakfast ideas

- Yogurt with fruit, and/or cinnamon, and/or nuts or seeds, and/or flax seed oil.
- Oatmeal with raisons, and/or nuts or seeds, and/or maple syrup, and/or cinnamon, and/or blueberries.
- Smoothies made with any combination of the following ingredients: yogurt, bananas, fruit in season, cinnamon, 100% juice, flax seed oil, optional protein powder or green super foods.
- Two eggs with rye bread and a dab of unsalted butter.
- Ancient grain cereal with greek yogurt or your selection of milk.

## Sample lunch ideas

- Green salad with any combination of the following ingredients:

any fruits or vegetables (preferably organic and locally grown), nuts and/or seeds with a home-made dressing that includes: onions, garlic, flax seed oil, balsamic vinegar, and maple syrup. You can include a piece of rye bread with hummus spread on the side.

- Any salad variation that includes healthy, whole foods, such as brown rice salads. But ensure that you are including a home-made, non-cream based dressing.
- Freshly made or canned tuna packed in water with salad.
- Ancient grain pita wrap with hummus or tofu spread

### Sample dinner ideas

- Grilled or oven-roasted salmon with lemon, dill topping, or sesame oil and cilantro. Have raw or lightly cooked in-season vegetables and a salad on the side.
- Brown rice, quinoa, or other ancient grain choices, mixed with vegetables and balsamic vinaigrette dressing.
- Home-made soups, stews or chilis made with fresh vegetables and limited salt. Include a salad on the side.
- Tofu fries with tamari sauce along with vegetables or a salad.
- Cabbage rolls made with rice, bulgur, cous cous or quinoa inside. Along with a salad with all the fixings!

### Sample snack ideas

- Fruit
- Trail mix
- Raw or lightly toasted nuts
- Dates, raisins, figs, apricots or other dried fruit (unsulphered)
- Fruit leather

- Apple sauce
- Raw vegetables
- Celery stuffed with hummus or nut butters
- Sandwiches on whole grains such as rye or spelt breads
- Home-made soup (not from a can)
- Blender drinks with 100% juices and fresh fruits (using only natural sugars)
- Frozen fruit popsicles
- Muffins, cookies, or bars made with natural sweeteners
- Popcorn (organic, unsalted)
- Puddings (made with natural or no sugars)
- Yogurts or apple (fruit) sauces (made with natural or no sugars). Add cinnamon for added flavour
- Whole grain crackers or rice cakes with nut butter or apple butter, rye crisps with spreads or corn chips with salsa.
- Ancient grain cereals or porridge with no added salt, sugars or preservatives.

### Sample day: Menu planning

*BREAKFAST*
- Nectarine (medium)
- Ancient grain cereal with rice, almond or cow's milk

*MORNING SNACK*
- Berries and yogurt

*LUNCH*
- Salad with home-made balsamic dressing
- Chicken breast

- One slice of rye bread
- Carrot and cucumber slices

*AFTERNOON SNACK*
- Prepared hummus
- Celery sticks

*DINNER*
- Steamed brown rice
- Green and yellow beans with mushrooms
- Grilled fish
- Salad (with home-made dressing)

### General tips for sample menu planning

- If you choose not to eat animal protein, simply substitute your favorite plant-based protein source for any of the suggested meat or fish items.
- To add savory flavor to dishes, consider using stocks and broths, fresh or dried herbs, wines, vinegars, ginger, garlic and onions rather than processed sauces or salt.
- Always have loads of vegetables cut and cleaned at all times.

**Lunch tip:** Start each meal off with a large salad made with an array of raw and cooked vegetables. Remember to emphasize dark greens and mix it up with varieties. Add healthy fats from whole food sources like nuts, seeds and avocados. Include your favorite beans or whole grains whenever you can. Fruit, such as berries, apples, pears, stone fruits and citrus also makes a delicious addition to salads.

**Snack tip:** Keep cut vegetables and fruit on hand for quick snacks. Prepare a fruit platter as soon as you get home from the grocery store and store in the fridge.

**Dinner tip:** Rethink your plate: eat your fill of vegetables and grains and if you eat animal products, use them with a light hand to accent a dish. With fish or chicken, emphasize healthier cooking methods such as baking, grilling, steaming, poaching and braising.

**Batch cooking** - Batch cooking is cooking a number of meals at once and freezing them for later use. This cooking strategy eases pressure, enhances healthy eating, and helps you naturally manage your weight. It also has the advantage of saving you prep time and money (as you buy products in bulk, and avoid take-out). It is such a healthy and efficient way to manage your diet because, by preparing meals in advance, in those times of last-minute meal decisions, you are pulling from your freezer, rather than your pocket-book and buying fast-food. When you do pull meals from the freezer, be sure to add foods like salads and fresh vegetables to your meal in order to add life force, enzymes and nutrients that might be lost from freezing. Batch cooking is the secret weapon to save time in the kitchen and make eating real food easy. Remember, you can make food ahead of time and have meals ready in the fridge to go for when your weekdays get really busy.

Freezer meals are entire meals prepped in advance, and then frozen for later use. They can either be completely cooked, so that all they need is thawing and reheating, or you can prepare most of the steps in advance, so that all that's left is cooking the meal. If you know you will eat that meal during the week, prepare it and store it in the fridge, making sure to note the date of first refrigeration on the container. Most home cooked foods can be frozen, but some foods are best eaten sooner rather than later or the texture will change if left in the freezer for too long. Always wrap food carefully to avoid freezer burn, but leave enough room for the foods to expand.

**Freeze:** Soups, sauces, shepherd's pie, stews or lasagna.


**Refrigerate:** Chicken or fish for on top of your salads. Hard boiled eggs, whole grain pasta, brown rice, roasted vegetables, roasted potatoes/sweet potatoes, or hummus.

*"If you don't find time for fitness, you better make time for being sick."*

— *Unknown*

Week seven of Mission Slim Possible! will allow you to explore how taking personal responsibility for your level of success on your Mission can drive positive change, both in your weight-balancing approach as well as in your life overall. This week I encourage you to step things up a notch, eliminate or minimize any self-pity or excuses and replace it with full active responsibility for your life and results. Try to plan and build workouts and active living into your life. Also, plan your nutrition for the week to help you on your Mission. Menu planning and preparation contributes to healthy eating and natural weight balancing. It's time to step it up a notch with tough love this week! Excuses and self-pity can deflate you on your Mission, it's time to take responsibility and accountability for your life.

# STAY ON TARGET

## MY WEEKLY CHECKLIST

- [x] Plan your week
- [x] Plan food
- [x] Plan workouts
- [x] Take responsibility
- [ ] _____
- [ ] _____
- [ ] _____
- [ ] _____
- [ ] _____
- [ ] _____
- [ ] _____
- [ ] _____
- [ ] _____
- [ ] _____
- [ ] _____
- [ ] _____
- [ ] _____
- [ ] _____

## MY WEIGHT THIS WEEK:

Began at:_____

Finished at:_____

Total weight loss:_____

## MY MEASUREMENTS THIS WEEK:

### BEGAN AT

Shoulders:_____

Chest:_____

Waist:_____

Hips:_____

### FINISHED AT

Shoulders:_____

Chest:_____

Waist:_____

Hips:_____

### DIFFERENCE/TOTAL INCHES LOST:

Shoulders:_____

Chest:_____

Waist:_____

Hips:_____

What really resonated for me this week?

_____

_____

_____

_____

_____

_____

_____

_____

_____

_____

What worked well for me this week?

_____

_____

_____

_____

_____

_____

_____

_____

_____

_____

_____

# WEEK EIGHT

# Psychology Management/Self-Coaching

The psychological relationship you have with food plays a huge roll on your Mission to slim. Banish cultural pressure, deprivation thinking and gain psychological control.

# Recreation Management

Become a morning exerciser and be energized for the day. Boost metabolism and fit your workouts in consistently.

# Nutrition Management

The psychology of being slim and healthy and how it relates to nutrition, food selection and control.

*"Learn from the past, set vivid, detailed goals for the future, and live in the only moment of time which you have any control: now."*

— *Denis Waitley*

# — WEEK EIGHT —

## Psychology Management/Self- Coaching

The psychological relationship and control you have with food plays a huge roll on your Mission to slim. Banish cultural pressure, deprivation thinking and gain psychological control.

Welcome to week eight of Mission Slim Possible! This week will allow you to gain psychological control, banish deprivation thinking, and improve your psychological relationship with nutrition and fitness while on your Mission to drive positive change. There is psychology behind being slim and healthy. In fact, as you can tell from this book, there is a huge section every single week addressing your psychology. Some might even go as far and say, the problem of weight management is associated with the lack of psychological control. Mission Slim

Possible is about taking back your psychological control and responsibility in you life to help drive you closer to your target! You are in control of that ideal person you have in your head! Now is the time to direct your food choices and feel empowered as a result.

There is a psychology behind being slim and healthy. The secret to losing weight and staying slim and healthy is to gain control of your life. Everyone has that point in their life when they feel they have hit a brick wall. For many people, losing control could mean gaining weight, becoming an alcoholic, starting smoking, or simply letting your workouts slide. Nutritionally, when you feel out of control of your life, you feel out of control of food and vise versa. There is one simple solution to this feeling: You need to get motivated to change! More specifically, I believe one of the major problem of weight management, is associated with the degree to which we lack psychological control. Once you realize this, you gain an understanding of what is needed to change and to be successful. You are in control of that ideal person you have in your head! Now is the time to direct your food choices and feel empowered as a result. With the idea of you directing your food choices, you will learn control and be able to manage food favorably for the rest of your life. It will help you with self-discovery, self-mastery, and self-regulation. This is the psychology of being slim and healthy - the mentality of managing weight. Healthy choices are essential. However, there is a major psychological component that needs to be addressed in order to be successful on all levels. If you want to manage your weight you need to manage your psychology. Your relationship with food mentally is just as important as the actual food you put into your body.

## What is deprivation thinking?

A state of deprivation means that you feel you are missing something, and the situation isn't comfortable. If you're deprived of something you feel a sense of lack or loss. Eating healthy is one of the biggest goals people make for themselves often. I can't help but to find it a bit funny, when people get upset they can't have that "treat" or they can't have that second serving because they are on a diet. The reason I find it funny, is that if they saw that food for what it really was, they would not be feeling deprived at all. If they were not on a crazy restriction diet, but rather eating natural, alive good quality foods, they would not feel deprived in any way. You don't need to feel deprived when you're losing weight. Deprivation can backfire when your on your Mission Slim Possible, because it causes you to feel like you are not enjoying the weigh loss process. But the process is amazing and every step and change is well worth every adjustment. Deprivation, in my opinion is a state of mind you can shift and change. People who believe healthy eating, active living and a strong mind is boring and bland, will start to feel deprived and not enjoy the process. However, by making smart choices every day, you can develop new eating habits, life habits and a high level of optimism, being on your Mission, simply is not deprivation but rather, a fantastic process that makes you happy.

## How deprivation is an illusion and holds us back from our target:

A common story people face when changing eating habits or being on a weight management program is the feeling of being deprived. With diets, for example, the attempt is to make people follow certain rules about certain foods in order to cut calories and lose weight. As your body seeks balance and becomes more aware, you realize that there are different parts of the mind that don't always agree with the strict program. One part of the mind follows the rules of the diet, while the other part of the mind reacts as if it were being deprived. And, as is the case with many diets, you really are depriving your body of adequate nutritional foods such as proteins and carbohydrates. But, those foods such as sugary and highly processed foods that are eliminated (and rightly so), trick your brain into thinking you are being deprived. These feelings of deprivation lead to cravings and a lack of control, and are the culprits that usually cause diets to fail. When you are nutritionally deprived of essential foods, this can lead to cravings and over-eating of the wrong foods, and ultimately weight gain.

The key to success then, is to manage your food so that you simply never feel deprived. The Mission Slim Possible program allows you to continue to consume all the healthy and nutritionally dense, whole foods so that you always feel satisfied. To gain power over your choices of how you treat your body entails getting power back from the voices and goals you have set. It becomes much easier to make changes in habits, such as eating, when you become aware of all the little habits that your mind has created. These are some common ways that we associate food with emotions and events:

- Food is success
- Food is reward
- Food is joy
- Food is relief from boredom
- Food is consolation
- Food is celebration
- Food is comfort, "eat it and you'll feel better"

**How the culture and society influences us on our Mission:**

A very important element to weight management is the pressure we get from the 'too-thin' imagery that society bombards us through the media. In most cases, the message we receive is that to be thin is synonymous with beauty, and this is neither realistic nor healthy. It is important to note that being overweight is not usually healthy, but slim can be a very specific definition for a body type. It is therefore important to remember that you need to establish your realistic image of what you want your success to look like, what slim and healthy means to you. Not what it looks like in the magazines, on celebrities etc. Once you establish that you can work diligently on changing your psychological relationship with foods. Be sure to clearly, and realistically, define what it means to be slim and healthy for you. Don't let cultural pressures, social events, unrealistic images, and hyper-exposure to food be your excuses for not reaching your goals.

**How to gain psychological control?**

I invite you to see food for what it really is and change your psychology around food. No deprivation, just the decision that you will feel, look and be a better person without that bag of chips, row of cookies, or block of cheese. Changing your mind-set is the backbone to reaching your target. You have a choice to use our culture and deprivation as excuses or you can change your mind and give yourself back the power. Gaining psychological control is about taking ownership of your goals and sticking to what you value and desire for your self.

*Change from being controlled by your food to being in control of your food choices.*

## Tips to gain control of your life:

- Accept that you life has gone off track and that change is needed
- Make mental images of the person you want to be.
- Write down a list of personality characteristics and traits of your 'ideal self'.
- Write down three goals you want to achieve soon.
- Be your ideal self for one day (observe how you feel).
- Add more and more days and become that person in your head.
- Create a weekly goal list.
- Write down ten strengths that you have and use them to your advantage.
- Get rid of negativity in your life.
- Remind yourself of the special person you are.
- Build your self-esteem.
- Establish daily priorities.
- Streamline your life.
- Cut back on unnecessary activities to free up time and energy.
- Make use of your travel time in the car (great time to learn).
- De-clutter your life, home and office.
- Know your limitations.
- Wake up earlier.
- Be more decisive and stick to your plan.
- Assess your idea of slim and healthy.
- Revisit your target and action plan on your Mission often.
- Focus on what is really important to you.
- Share the load of responsibility; delegate and/or ask for help.

Taking control of your life is essential to managing your life. Gaining and maintaining control over what happens in your life is never straightforward, but by following these tips you will be well on your way to improving the amount of control that you do have, which will ultimately make you happier and more successful on your Mission.

**Why gaining control is important on your Mission?**

By directing your food choices you will realize weight balancing is a process about making decisions that are really important to you, and what you are willing to do to achieve the goals you set for yourself. This is the psychology behind your weight management efforts – it's not about deprivation, rather it's about focus and deciding what you want. Gaining control is empowering. To succeed, you can focus on:

- Your goals
- Your Mission
- Your target
- Your decisions
- Your weight
- Your mini targets

- Your success
- Your health
- Your accomplishments
- Your pride
- Your passion
- Your energy

*Remember: "strong and healthy is the new skinny."*

You control what you put into your mouth and you make the decisions. When you decide that you are not deprived and that your goals are much more important than those cravings, it will bring forth liberation. This is gaining control and taking ownership for your life and reality.

**It's time for self-coaching and inner reflection:**

Take time to answer and work through these questions in your journal to help keep you focused and on a clear path towards your goals. By taking action you will bring your goals into your life. These self-coaching questions will help clarify what you need to have accomplished this week.

**Self-Coaching Questions**

- What needs to happen each day this week?
- What are my priorities this week?
- How will these action steps help me get closer to my goals?
- In the next week my complete focus will be on?
- My direction is clear to me because...?
- I am willing to commit to...?
- What might success look like to me for this week?
- What resonated and stood out to me from the program and what impact will it have on me this week?
- I deserve this because...?
- I am thrilled with myself because…?
- Why is it important for me to take action and follow my goals this week?

# — NOTES —

*"Exercise should be regarded as a
tribute to the heart."*

— *Gene Tunney*

# — WEEK EIGHT —

## Recreation Management

Become a morning exerciser and get energized for the day. Boost metabolism and fit workouts in consistently.

Ben Franklin said it well, "Early to bed and early to rise make a man healthy, wealthy and wise." It applies to women of course too. Are you one of those people that will wake up long before the sun has shown its presence? Or, do you leave just enough time in the morning to roll out of bed, shower, and grab a cup of coffee en route to work? If you are the type of person that could sleep all day or is sluggish to rise in the morning, there are a ton of great benefits to waking up early.

## The benefits of waking up early:

This confession will come as no surprise to my friends and family, most of whom have spent many mornings avoiding me until I get my morning tea. People often ask me, "do you spring out of bed?" For years I've tried to be one of 'them', those chipper, cheerful people who rise effortlessly and early. Even though I am not naturally a morning person, I aspire to be one. I do most of my best work in the early hours of the day, anywhere from 6 a.m. to 9 a.m. Here are my top reasons to wake up early from my experience and those of my clients over the years.

- Greet the day first thing
- Don't miss out on anything and you get a head start
- Activate your metabolism early
- Chance to plan your day
- Amazing start to the day
- You become more proactive and productive
- You are more alert and get things done effectively
- Sleep better at night
- Eliminate rush and stress
- Gives you a feeling of more time and peace
- Quietude and enjoy stillness
- The morning is peaceful
- Sunrise is gorgeous
- Calm
- Extra time for exercise and being active
- Increase productivity in your life
- You'll be similar to many of the great achievers
- Work toward your life goals consistently

## The benefits of being a morning exerciser:

**Better impact on your body:** Your body responds well to a workout when you are fresh and well rested. So it makes sense that after a good night sleep is an optimal time to get your body in motion.

Exercising early in the morning "jump starts" your metabolism, keeping it elevated for hours, sometimes for up to 24 hours! As a result, you'll be burning more calories all day long—just because you exercised in the morning.

Exercising in the morning energizes you for the day—not to mention that gratifying feeling of virtue you have knowing you've done something disciplined and good for you.

**Prioritize:** We all have good intentions and so often our PLAN to work out gets put on the sidelines. Morning workouts make exercise a priority before the list of things you need to do during the day take over.

**Develops personal discipline:** Getting up early requires discipline and with this discipline comes success.

**Achievement:** Success and the feeling of achievement will help you build confidence. It feels so good when you are accomplishing your goals. By setting good habits and working out early daily, you are achieving a goal of active living.

**You have more time:** When the kids and others are still sleeping, waking up early gives you more time to yourself.

**Focus:** An early morning workout will free up the rest of your day and allow you to focus on the things you need to achieve. Studies have shown that exercise significantly increases mental acuity—a benefit that lasts four to ten hours after your workout ends.

Exercising in the a.m. means you get to harness that brainpower, instead of wasting it while you're snoozing. How many times have you planned on working out after work when something better comes along or you get too tired so you just go home?

By getting up early, you have fewer schedule conflicts and are less likely to miss out on any fun later in the day or get distracted. Instead you are guaranteed your work out.

**Great attitude:** Exercise makes you feel better, so by doing your exercise first thing in the morning you set yourself up for a great day. Your body produces "feel good" hormones when you workout which help relieve stress and make you feel happier.

By getting your exercise in first thing, you have a better diet all day and you will approach your food choices differently. You are more likely to continue your motivation through out the day.

### How to get started being a morning exerciser:

To start, go to bed earlier. I suggest going to bed earlier, even if you don't think you'll sleep, and read while in bed. If you're really tired, you just might fall asleep much sooner than you think. Start slowly, by waking just fifteen to thirty minutes earlier than usual. Get used to this for a few days. Then cut back another fifteen minutes. Do this gradually until you get to your goal time. You don't need to make drastic changes. Try not to hit snooze and get up right away when your alarm goes off. Don't allow yourself to rationalize going back to bed. Just force yourself to go out of the room to the bathroom. By the time you have brushed your teeth, washed hands and face, you'll be awake enough to face the day. Have a routine, a good reason established and create a plan. If you don't have something planned or something important to do in the morning with the extra time you have from waking up early, you'll find yourself lacking motivation to get out of bed. Establish a morning routine that you start as soon as you wake up. If you allow your brain to talk you out of getting up early, you'll never do it. Don't make getting back in bed an option. Make waking up early a reward. Find something that's pleasurable for you and allow yourself to do it as part of your morning routine. My favourite thing to wake up to is my morning tea and watching the birds outside, while I let me dog out. I take a deep breath and enjoy the fresh quiet air. Get a jump start on your day and take advantage of all that extra time.

With all the craziness of kids, work and life, it can be particularly challenging to make the time to exercise. But doing your workout in the morning is a wonderful way to create positive consistent routines and provides many additional benefits as outlined in this chapter. The good news is that you get to decide the best time for you to exercise based upon your personal goals, schedule and lifestyle. Ideally, you will pick a time that you are able to stick with consistently and make part of your daily or weekly schedule. Exercise at any time of day can provide your mind and body with a life-changing boost. Just make an effort to be consistent and don't let excuses stop you from being the best you can be!

*"Nothing tastes as good as being skinny feels"*

— *Kate Moss*

# — WEEK EIGHT —

## Nutrition Management

The psychology of being slim and healthy and how it relates to cravings, trigger foods and control.

We have all experienced hunger, but what makes food cravings different from being hungry and how much psychological control do we have over these cravings. These cravings can pose a serious health threat and can be damaging on our Mission to be slim. For example, food cravings have been shown to elicit over eating episodes, which can lead to extra un-wanted calories and feelings of guilt and shame.

### What are food cravings?

When you are looking to make healthier food choices, understanding cravings is an essential component of staying on track. The key to understanding cravings is listening to your body. You want to clarify if your body is telling you it needs something, or is your mind telling you it wants something. As I mentioned earlier on the Mission, people are often undernourished, despite the fact that they may be overweight. Poor food choices, from over consumption of processed foods, can be largely to blame for this debt. Cravings can come from a place of malnutrition. Here lies the real paradox, feeling compelled to eat more and more of a substance that is not good for you and not providing you what you need, won't fix the problem. What your body really needs probably, are leafy greens and other nutrient dense vegetables, healthy fats, and water. Most of the time cravings are actually "wants." Why do we get intense desires to eat certain foods? Since food is essential to survival, and unlike any other addiction, it is a built-in safety mechanism and normal for us to feel that on a day-to-day basis. Hunger is built in, but cravings are created by our minds. The most common cravings or 'wants' are for things that are sweet, salty, and savory. You can use your cravings or wants to help make better choices.

Psychological scientists Eva Kemps and Marika Tiggemann of Flinders University, Australia, review the latest research on food cravings and how they may be controlled. Their research revealed that we may have more psychological control over cravings than we think. Though the exact cause of specific food cravings is difficult to pinpoint, many doctors and nutritionists alike believe that they develop as a result of a complex medley of biochemical processes, life experiences and a variety of hormonal and emotional factors. Likely most food cravings are actually food "wants", the good news about these "wants", we have control over them. If you are craving high calorie diet busting foods devoid of nutrition, you are probably responding to a craving rather than hunger. What is the difference? A craving is based on your psychology; hunger is rooted in your biology. When you are hungry, any food could really satisfy you, but cravings are specific, intense desires to eat a particular food. Your secret on your Mission, is to differentiate between the two. The only thing that can stop a food craving is to substitute foods for other healthy options, distract your self, use portion control, or give into the craving. Since we know that cravings are largely psychologically based, all we have to do is gain psychological control! Easy, right? Let's take a look at food triggers and addiction first.

### What are trigger foods and how they relate to addiction?

Eating helps to build our bodies, keep us healthy, replenish used vitamins and minerals and food is a vital source to provide fuel. This is the common focus for many people. Unfortunately, for others, food can cause 'perceived', uncontrollable cravings that manifests as an addiction and leads to over consumptions of sugars and/or carbohydrates that leads to consequences. Many of my clients claim that potato chips are one of their triggers and they cannot stop at one; they will consume large quantities of chips even when they are full. Trigger foods are the foods that prompt chain eating that very much mimics addiction. Food addiction affects an individual physically, emotionally, spiritually and socially. Food addicts gain pleasure from thinking about the food they crave, and excessively eat the food, often not even aware of the pattern and the improper eating habits become a way of life. The Sooner you realize you need help with your food addiction, the easier it is to gain psychological control. Either way if you are addicted to food or have severe or strong uncontrollable cravings for certain foods, you are ready for the next steps to isolate and remove your trigger foods and addiction. Identifying your trigger foods, or foods that trigger addictive behaviours, you are one step closer to overcoming food addiction and gaining psychological control.

**Some symptoms of possible food addiction or excessive cravings:**

- Inability to control cravings for food or to control amount of food that is eaten.
- Trying many different weight loss or diet programs but still excessively consuming food.
- Feeling ashamed about your weight. Feeling depressed or sad about your weight or self-image.
- Eating when upset or depressed or eating as a reward for a job well done.
- Eating behind closed doors to prevent others from seeing what you are eating or how much.
- Avoiding social interactions because you don't feel like you look good enough or have clothes that fit correctly due to your eating habits.
- Marked increase in the amounts of food consumed over time.
- Eating when emotionally upset or depressed.
- Stealing food from others or obsessing over food.

The good news is, you don't have to be stuck in this 'victim to food' state you have the power to gain control and take back your life. The key is in isolating the trigger foods and gaining psychological control.

## How trigger foods affect you on your Mission:

In a sense, we are all addicted to food. Think about how it feels when you are not able to eat and you are hungry. You start to crave food, your stomach makes noises and hunger becomes increasingly physically and emotionally uncomfortable. The longer the cravings for food from hunger go on for, the more intense the need to eat becomes, eating becomes the most important thing for you to do. This is a natural healthy process built into your biology to keep you healthy and nourished. The problem starts when your cravings and trigger foods take over this natural process, causing you to gain weight from excessive calories consumption. Trigger foods can be like an addiction, they cause excessive eating, weight gain and ill health. You can't stop at just one. Once you have one, you end up eating an entire row, box or bag. Like alcohol or any other drug addiction, food addiction has side-effects and can have quite an impact on your life. Obesity, weight-gain, lifestyle changes, social implications and health risks are just a few of the possible side-effects. The problem begins when we have this feeling towards food that does not support our health and weight management attempts. What happens is we tend to give trigger foods the ability to take over and control our decisions and it is time to gain back that control.

## How to idetify your trigger (addictive) food:

By identifying the foods that have controlled and influenced you before and by isolating the foods that have sabotaged your Mission attempts in the past, is the key to gain control. Like an addict to alcohol, just admitting the addiction is the first step towards healing and gaining control. I often suggest that you make a list of all your favorite foods. Chances are your trigger foods are on this list. I know mine are cookies, chips and cheese. These foods have sabotaged my Mission attempts in the past and are definitely trigger foods for me. If I don't start with these foods, I don't have a problem. Once you have the list, do you notice a pattern? Have any of these foods sabotaged your previous weight balancing attempts? Ask yourself and answer honestly the following questions about your list of foods:

- Have you told yourself, "I will just have one," or "I will have just a little"?
- When you see it, do you crave it?
- Do you feel sluggish or fatigued from overeating?
- Do you have withdrawal symptoms like agitation and anxiety when you cut out certain foods?
- Do you feel out of control when you start with this certain food?
- Do you keep eating this food despite significant emotional and/ or physical problems associated from eating it?
- Do you eat it even when you are not even hungry?
- When you see it, do you crave it?
- Do you try and explain or justify purchasing the foods?
- Have you eaten it instead of a meal?
- Do you always eat it in certain situations?
- Do you try hard to give it up, but find it hard to stay away?
- When you gained weight before, were you eating this food?

If you answered 'yes' to any of these questions, then you probably identified your trigger foods, the foods that have sabotaged your Mission to be healthy and slim in the past. Look at your list, take a strong hard look at it. Don't leave anything out as a result of denial. This is your special personal list now! Know what foods are your trigger foods. This is your personal secret to losing all your unwanted pounds. It is time to gain control. Another way to isolate some of what could be your trigger foods, is to start a food journal. Observe your selection for the entire week. Look for numerous repetitions of food choices, high quantity of food, and also look into the foods that you may have "forgotten" to add to your food journal.

**How to gain psychological control over food selection:**

Now that you have identified the foods that are your trigger to overeating, these are the foods that you need to choose to eliminate from your everyday food choices. Just by identifying the triggers that have sabotaged your Mission in the past or caused weight gain or lack of control, you are on the path to gaining control. Remember, these foods have done nothing good for you in the past and have actually contributed to your struggles. It is important to see these trigger foods for what they really are to you. They are your enemy and cause weight gain, poor health, fatigue and stress. They are: Not treats, not goodies, not rewards, they add weight on, they damage your self-confidence, they decrease your energy levels, they limit your clothing selection, they add on pounds, they make your clothing tight, they make you stressed, they decrease energy levels. They are: Not comfort, not a treat at all, they make you sad, they make the scale increase, they decrease your desire to socialize, they are actually your enemy. I usually put a picture of myself, where I am not pleased with the way I look in the photo, and I tape it onto the cookie jar, bag of chips, and cheese. It amazes me, when I make the direct connection; that is what those trigger foods do to me. I can clearly see the weight they put on and the effect it has on my Mission. These foods have a price to pay for eating them – we'll have to wear these trigger foods, quit literally! Like drugs, trigger foods have a destructive effect on behavior, causing us to decrease control, despite our best intentions and determinations. It's time to gain control and isolate our trigger foods. Gain control and eliminate these foods entirely.

*We can't have it both ways; we either choose our Slim Mission, or the trigger food, it is entirely up to you.*

It all comes back to you again. It is entirely up to you as an individual; only you can choose what is most important to you. You can trade off one or more of your trigger foods to stay on your Mission and be that slim, healthy person you always wanted to be or you can choose to accept limitations in exchange for feeling awful in your tight clothes having low energy and poor health. When you decide to choose wellness, the price you will pay will be feelings of health, energy, slimness, pride, increased self-esteem, wellness and a wonderful desire to  socialize and wear nice clothing!  In order to connect with your food in a new manner you need to change your mindset and see food for what it really is.

*By gaining psychological control and directing your food choices you accept your responsibility and can stay true to your mission.*

The bottom line is that you have more control over your health and food choices than you may think or believe. Control is the state of being cognitively skillful or aware. We have a built in mechanism that controls the operation of our bodily functions and that is automatic, but we sometimes let the outside world take over control of the choices we can make. Hunger is not a signal we want to ignore, however, food cravings are definitely something we need to monitor. There are some trigger foods that can be troublesome and require our special recognition and attention. You can actually shift towards the healthy, optimistic and goal-oriented mindset by identifying the trigger foods that have controlled you in the past; the foods that have sabotaged your weight-loss attempts or have even caused weight gain in the first place. Just by acknowledging, taking back control on food choices, and seeing food for what it really is, you take back responsibility and ownership for your life!

### How to stop food cravings and gain psychological control:

I bet you want to stop eating unhealthy, tempting, calorie filled foods. If you do frequently experience intense food cravings, which are a hindrance for whatever reason, then there are ways of reducing them.

### Try these additional tips to halt food cravings and gain psychological control:

- Eat regularly
- Choose foods low on the Glycemic Index
- Restrict sugar intake
- Reduce salt intake
- Identify your trigger food: know what you want to avoid
- Know the difference between your healthy food and treats
- Avoid processed foods
- Exercise
- Take yourself away from the food
- Remove yourself from situations that promote trigger food eating

- Think about the negatives involved
- Eat an alternative to your craving
- Drink lots of water
- Distract yourself from the food you crave
- Be aware of the benefits of avoiding the food you crave
- Put the food you crave out of sight or remove it from your possession
- Connect with your mind and reclaim your power
- Practice saying NO
- Brush your teeth
- Meditate and do yoga
- Connect to your goals

There is a psychology behind being slim and healthy. The secret to losing weight and staying slim and healthy is to gain control of your life. When you are looking to make healthier food choices, understanding cravings is an essential component of staying on track. By gaining psychological control and directing your food choices you accept your responsibility and can stay true to your mission. Get a jump start on your day, wake up early and take advantage of all that extra time. We can't have it both ways; we either choose our Slim Mission, or the trigger foods can take over, the choice is entirely up to you.

# STAY ON TARGET

## MY WEEKLY CHECKLIST

- [x] Gain control of your life
- [x] Understand cravings
- [x] Accept your role
- [x] Get a jump start on your day
- [x] Wake up early
- [x] Identify trigger foods
- [ ] 
- [ ] 
- [ ] 
- [ ] 
- [ ] 
- [ ] 
- [ ] 
- [ ] 
- [ ] 
- [ ] 
- [ ] 

## MY WEIGHT THIS WEEK:

Began at:_____

Finished at:_____

Total weight loss:_____

## MY MEASUREMENTS THIS WEEK:

### BEGAN AT

Shoulders:_____

Chest:_____

Waist:_____

Hips:_____

### FINISHED AT

Shoulders:_____

Chest:_____

Waist:_____

Hips:_____

## DIFFERENCE/TOTAL INCHES LOST:

Shoulders:_____

Chest:_____

Waist:_____

Hips:_____

What really resonated for me this week?

_____

_____

_____

_____

_____

_____

_____

_____

_____

_____

_____

What worked well for me this week?

_____

_____

_____

_____

_____

_____

_____

_____

_____

_____

_____

_____

# WEEK NINE

## Psychology Management/Self-Coaching

Find happiness and acceptance of your self, while on your Mission. Learn the benefits of managing your expectations and stopping the tendency to compare.

## Recreation Management

Effective ways to lose belly fat with these tips and workouts for a flatter stomach. Try some abdominal blasting challenges!

## Nutrition Management

By keeping your blood sugar levels under control, you can lose fat, regulate mood, and boost energy levels. Eating a lot of fiber can help you to lose weight and regulate blood sugar levels.

*"If you paint in your mind a picture of bright and happy expectations, you put yourself into a condition conducive to your goal."*

— *Norman Vincent Peale*

# — WEEK NINE —

## Psychology Management/Self- Coaching

Find happiness and acceptance of your self, while on your Mission. Learn the benefits of managing your expectations and stopping the tendency to compare.

Welcome to week nine of Mission Slim Possible! This week will allow you to find happiness and acceptance of your self, while on your Mission. You will learn the benefits and tools of managing expectations, along with effective ways to lose belly fat for a flatter stomach. Finally, by keeping your blood sugar levels under control, you will see how you can lose fat, regulate mood, and boost energy levels. We also discuss how eating a lot of fiber can help you to lose weight and regulate blood sugar levels. Remember: There are two ways to be happy: Improve your reality or lower your expectations. Lowering your expectation simply is not an option, when you have selected Mission Slim Possible!

**What are expectations? Can they help us or hinder us?**

We all have expectations in our lives - what we want out of life and who we want to become. I believe one of the solutions to happiness lies within the management of our expectations of people, ourselves and our circumstances. When we have realistic expectations, we can never be disappointed. Healthy expectations drive motivation and standards. Healthy expectations are realistic. Having realistic expectations allow us to accept the flaws, or downfalls, in ourselves, and in others. The question becomes, do expectations help us or hinder us?

The key to our well-being and happiness is not to lower our expectations. It is the ability to interpret unexpected negative outcomes in a positive way and to make our expectations realistic. Once we realize that our expectations cannot change people, and our expectations for ourselves are perhaps too high, the better off we will be. An unfortunate pitfall of having high expectations in certain circumstances is that we prevent ourselves from enjoying the experience altogether. The pressure becomes too great and we then lack a level of self-love and acceptance. You can see the dilemma here. Too high levels of expectations of ourselves, puts pressure and sets us up for disappointment. While lowering expectations seems counter productive along our Mission. If you feel this way in your life, you need to readjust your expectations. Do not go into into situations with unrealistic expectations; instead, go into them with an open mind. This will allow you to fully immerse yourself without the pressure of living up to preconceived notions. When you have unrealistic notions for people, or yourself, you place yourself at a high risk of getting disappointed and hurt.

Is there a paradoxical issue when it comes to expectations? In fact there is. If you have high expectations, you can often end up disappointed, but the paradox is if you don't have high expectations, you may not try as hard in order to accomplish a goal. If you expect your body to be "perfect", you will often be disappointed in yourself. However, if you don't aspire to have a fit, strong and healthy body, then motivation to reach your weight management goals may not be strong. So, the negative side of expectation is when your expectation is unrealistic, which, can turn people into perfectionists, which is far from a healthy lifestyle or way to live. Expect what you can, reach for your goals and be aware of the fact that sometimes life throws you a curve ball. Try to remain confident while maintaining positive aspirations; just remember not to make these aspirations so high that they are impractical or unreachable. Setting subjective expectations high or low has objective consequences.

*The key to our well-being is not to lower expectations. It is the ability to interpret unexpected negative outcomes in a more positive way and make sure expectations were realistic to begin with.*

### Why does the ability to managing expectations become important?

Simply put, expectations are those wishes or desires of what we expect to accomplish or achieve in ourselves or in others. If you expect to be a doctor, you have to be willing to sacrifice at least eight years of your life to achieve that goal. If you expect to be an athlete, you have to train hours to achieve the level of fitness required. If you expect a perfect husband that does laundry, you may be setting yourself up for disappointment. Managing expectations of our own, and as well as the expectations of others in our lives can creates breathing room for our experiences, allowing us to live with more certainty and calm and encouraging less reactivity and avoiding upset. We all have expectations of people, events, our bodies and the restaurants we eat at, for example. Most of the time our expectations live below our subconscious mind and we do not know we had the expectation until we are either happily surprised or disappointed. Managing expectations with people does take time, however it will help you when expectations are not met. It is not about lowering expectations so that you are always happy with the outcome, nor is it having such high expectations that you are constantly disappointed. The balance and the managing of your expectations is what will become crucial to your happiness.

*"There are two ways to be happy: Improve your reality or lower your expectations" -Unknown*

### Learn lessons when expectations are not met:

Unmet expectations are those expectations that collide with reality, leaving you feeling upset and angry. If you expected to lose 10 pound in one week, you have set yourself up for disappointment. It's important to remember that sometimes you are going to lose, or fall short of your expectation and when that happens, you have to exercise self-control. The take-home message here is that there are no guarantees in love, in work, or in life. So, exercising self-control when you are faced with disappointment or the unexpected will allow you to be gentle on yourself and others and reevaluate. You have the ability to work hard and smart, simultaneously. The key is balancing your level of expectations and ability to be flexible and accepting. The successful management of expectations requires realistic life choices and recognition that sometimes things are not going to work the way you expected. The choice then is how do you deal with this new reality? Learn from the unmet expectation. Evaluate your expectation and level of realism. Evaluate your behaviour and the behaviour of others around the disappointment, or unmet expectation, and decide where adjustment needs to be made. Ask yourself these questions: Did you communicate your expectation to others? Did your actions support your expectation for yourself? Is the expectation realistic? Do you need to adjust your level of expectations?

**Communicating your expectations is the key:**

We often expect people—our friends, our family, our co-workers and sometimes the public—to be mind readers. "Don't they know what I'm going through? Don't they know what I'm thinking and feeling?" "Doesn't he know I like floors vacuumed every week?" Well, no. If you do not communicate your needs and wants and explain yourself, you will be disappointed. Ask and you shall receive. Power is not something that is given. You need to ask for it, "I want that time to work out," "I want to be treated with respect," "I want to eat somewhere healthy." At the very least, depending on the response, you will know where you stand and then can make strategic moves to improve your situation.

**Talk about other's expectations of you:**

Many people do not manage the expectations of others well. Few people start a new job, project, team or customer relationship and actually take the time to sit together and talk about the expectations of all parties. What do I expect from the job, my boss, the company, the customer? What does the company expect from me? For example, I remember a time I was really angry with my husband for going biking and leaving me all day with the kids. There is a clearly unmet need and level of unmet expectation at play. My expectations was that my husband help me with the kids, ask me to go biking with him, or communicate what his plans might be for the day. His expectations were very different; it was his day off and he believed it was his time to go biking. He had the expectation that I would look after the kids and so he could go on with his day and get his exercise. We all see the inherent problem with this scenario. There was no clear communication on what each other's expectations were for that day. Had we sat down the night before and gone over how we wanted to spend the weekend, all the anger, frustration and resentment may have been avoided. It is a good idea, then, to discuss your expectations with others and also have their expectations of you expressed. Or to put it another way, if you notice you are angry, upset or frustrated, then look at your unmet expectations.

*Managing expectations is about eliminating the gap between what we expect and what happens.*

**Personal expectations and acceptance:**

We can apply this same process to our own unmet expectations of ourselves. Take time to voice your upset, either in your inner dialogue, via writing, or by speaking this out with a willing listener such as your coach. Look at what you were expecting, and then distinguish the gap. Managing expectations is about eliminating the gap between what we expect and what happens. For example, my client Brenda (name changes for privacy reasons) expected to lose ten pounds before her friend's wedding. She did not lose the expected weight and as a result, felt terrible in her dress and not at all excited to go to the wedding. Look closely at the gap between what she wanted and what actually happened. Was it a realistic expectation in the first place? Did she make achievable action plans? What did she actually do to try and meet that expectation? Turns out, Brenda expected this weight loss to happen in two weeks. She had deadlines and stress at work and as a result, she failed to change her eating habits, drink water, or attempt to fit workouts into her busy schedule. Sound familiar? Yes, life gets in the way sometimes. So when I asked her to identify the gap, she realized she could have reframed her expectation to a more realistic expectation of being active for the next two weeks. She said it would have removed pressure and disappointment that caused her more stress. She would have stayed committed to her walking and workouts without the pressure to drop pounds.

On a personal level, managing expectations can be as simple as a reframing. For example, as a Life Coach, the expectation that I set for myself was to have my first book completed, marketed and promoted within a year. When I started to write my first book in April 2008, I had not done enough research, training or work for this to happen. To build this unrealistic time-frame or expectation around the completion of the book lead only to disappointment. The strategy I used in this instance was to reframe my expectations to one of enjoying the writing process and knowing the content would help people upon completion. Not only did that remove the pressure, I managed to enjoy the process of reaching my goals. I reframed my expectation from focusing on time and deadlines to focusing on the quality of work and the enjoyment of the process. With this pressure removed, I was more creative, relaxed about my writing and was far more productive, allowing me to reach the goal of completing a good quality book that will help people.

If you are living with constant disappointment, I encourage you to sit down with a pen and paper and make a list of your expectations. This will allow you to look at how you manage your expectations. The list might be considerably long (no wonder we often feel disappointed or like a failure!). Sometimes we set an impossible number of tasks and goals to live up to. Now, with this list, begin to reframe these expectations, without lowering your standards. You do this by making sure you're still on target with your goals, but remove the unrealistic pressure around your expectations for yourself. When you do this, you will feel a sense of pressure release and happiness, and often, you will be able to meet and exceed many of your new expectations! Have a look at your own expectations. Observe the areas in your life where you are frustrated and upset. Observe the areas where your family, spouse or co-workers are upset. Learn to be a master of managing expectations. You will know when you are doing this because you will be happy, excited and have a sense of ease.

**Practicing Acceptance:**

Acceptance is an amazing trait that needs to be actively worked toward to help us through unmet expectations. When things do not work out the way we had planned, it is much more beneficial to realize that is how life works rather than becoming frustrated at the situation. It isn't easy to forget about things that you are disappointed with; like your lack of going to the gym this week or that you had over-indulged with sweets, but you can stop suffering and practice acceptance. Now, I am not saying it is okay to do these when you are trying very hard to lose weight, but I am suggesting that you move on from dwelling on this disappointment. Accept that the event has happened. Learn what you can from the event. Look for the gap between your expectations and reality. Reframe your expectations. Problem solve for a new approach. Acceptance is not about a passive resignation to the situation. Accept the situation, acknowledge the problem, and then consciously correct the situation through acceptance. Once you start becoming mindful of your tendencies, it's crucial that you don't judge yourself. Practice acceptance and embrace who you are. Become mindful, observe your thoughts, and breathe. Acceptance can be hard, but it's certainly possible.

### Tips for practicing acceptance and self-love:

**Compare yourself to yourself and not others:** We all have the tendency to compare ourselves to others. We often let other people get to us. We get stuck in comparing this with that, me with you, him with her, this job with that job, or this car to that car. Comparing yourself to others doesn't motivate you to do more or to be better; instead it makes you feel like you'll never be good enough. Comparing ourselves with others can be damaging to happiness and self-esteem. Why is comparing damaging? Society often projects flawless skin, big eyes, full lips, small nose, white teeth, smooth and shiny hair, curvy, slim, fit bodies, and designer clothes for women - and they portray them as being happy. They portray men with six pack abs, flawless skin, strong muscles and designer clothes as well. And guess what? He's happy too! Marketing and Advertising in the form of images from magazines, television, movies, and photos, for example are extremely effective in being able to brainwash viewers and readers into believing they should look a certain way, act a certain way, be a certain someone, when in reality every single one of us is different and SHOULD stay that way!

Comparing yourself to others, especially celebrities, and thinking you should look that way is going to throw out your self-esteem and flaw your thinking. Those images we see regularly are completely fake and unrealistic! There will always be those who are 'better looking' than you, and those who are 'worse looking' than you. Comparison takes you nowhere, wastes energy and time and puts you in a negative place.

**Let go of comparison and reveal your greatness.** Being present and limiting the tendencies to compare can dramatically reduce stress and increase happiness. Choose to only compare yourself to yourself. In other words, compare your week results with last week results. Just keep becoming a better and better version of yourself. Use this method of positive version of comparing, to propel you forward toward your target.

**Focus on yourself and only you:** Take action! Instead of comparing yourself to others, focus on what you are achieving on a personal level. Write out the five qualities you like best about yourself, than write out what you value most in your life. Begin to create a list of adjectives that describe you - at least 25 positive words about your greatness.

**Stop yourself from comparing right away:** Whenever you find yourself comparing, think of some of the adjectives that describe YOU. When you hear your 'inner-coach' or 'inner-voice' telling you what you haven't done right, turn down the volume on it and turn up the volume to hear the voice that knows the TRUTH about who you are and how you add value to the world. Recognize that comparing yourself to others is a bad habit.

**Notice good things and good habits:** Tony DiCicco, coach of the US Women's Soccer team, wrote a book called, "Catch Them Being Good". He pointed out that if you get in the habit of noticing good things, even in yourself, you'll notice more good things. You'll communicate positive expectations more often, and be able to notice great things in yourself and others and be less likely to compare. Ask yourself a new question: "What is going right?" or "What is working?" Begin to notice all the things, no matter how small, that are working well.

**Keep an evidence journal:** Keep an 'evidence journal' and each day write down everything (I do mean everything!) that is positive and working. You can choose to notice what you do that is good and that you can be proud of, no matter how small it may seem. Each day keep a log of what you are grateful for about YOU. Acknowledge five things each and every day that you did well.

**Compliment yourself regularly:** Each day, compliment yourself on something you did that you feel good about. Notice your small successes and let compliments others give you flow into your bones. Really take in those compliments others give you and make sure you give yourself credit too.

**Recognize everyone is different and unique:** People are born to be different and unique - no two people are the same. We will always have room for improvement, nobody is flawless or perfect, so keep an open mind and awareness that everyone is beautiful in his own way and that everyone has his own insecurities. Try to focus on what is unique and special about you personally and it will ease the pressure and stress that comparison can create.

**Make changes for yourself and only yourself:** If you feel you need self-improvement in some way and you have set yourself an attainable goal, go for it. If you believe that you really need change, do it now. Be sure that you're doing it because it will make you happier, rather than impressing somebody else. Don't do it because you're comparing yourself to others and you feel you don't measure up. Do it for yourself. Make sure your goals are for you and you alone. Self- improvement almost always makes us feel better about ourselves and changes our focus off of comparing and onto goals.

*Keep up the amazing work...*

**It's time for self-coaching and inner reflection:**

Take time to answer and work through these questions in your journal to help keep you focused and on a clear path towards your goals. By taking action you will bring your goals into your life. These self-coaching questions will help clarify what you need to have accomplished this week.

### Self-Coaching Questions

- What needs to happen each day this week?
- What are my priorities this week?
- How will these action steps help me get closer to my goals?
- In the next week my complete focus will be on?
- My direction is clear to me because...?
- I am willing to commit to...?
- What might success look like to me for this week?
- What resonated and stood out to me from the program and what impact will it have on me this week?
- I deserve this because...?
- I am thrilled with myself because…?
- Why is it important for me to take action and follow my goals this week?

# — NOTES —

*"I have flabby thighs, but fortunately my stomach covers them."*

— Joan Rivers

# — WEEK NINE —

## Recreation Management

Effective ways to lose belly fat with these tips and workouts for a flatter stomach. Try some abdominal blasting challenges!

What is the best strategy to banish belly fat? Is it as simple as adding certain foods to your diet and doing particular exercises? Having flat and toned abdominals is one of the most desired attributes people have for themselves. Many people struggle with a stubborn midsection and it isn't just simply a magical diet and a special workout that is going to do the trick, but rather a combination approach. According to American statistics, 90% of adults in the U.S. are not happy with their abdominal muscle tone and they would gladly have a flatter stomach or lose that stomach fat altogether.

Belly fat is not only unflattering, it is also linked to many health problems, such as bloating, heartburn, diabetes, heart disease, stroke and many others. The great news is that getting a flat abdomen and even those six-pack abs are not as difficult as many people may think. To lose stomach fat, you need to change your diet and exercise habits. It is not just about doing sit ups until you are blue in the face and exhausted.

### Tips to lose that belly fat:

- Lose weight - You have to lose weight or decide to lose a certain amount of weight to rid the belly of fat that is hiding your abdominal muscles. The entire Natural Weight Balancing Program will be already helping you in this department. This is not going to happen overnight though; you will definitely need to lose some excess weight if you have it, before you can lose that belly fat.

- Drink water - It is always a good idea to carry water with you everywhere you go and stay well hydrated. Water makes you feel fuller, energetic and prevents you from over-indulging. It prevents you from drinking other options that can bloat you. Cut out soda and sugary beverages. A serving of soda or iced tea contains a lot of extra calories that we don't need. Many calories come from high fructose corn syrup, which, as you now know, wreak havoc on our blood sugar levels and end up turning into stored belly fat. Studies have shown that if you are thirsty, you will also eat more. So before your meals, get in the habit of having a glass of water and wait a few minutes and you will be amazed how your portion size will change.

- Work It Out -  You don't have to do endless crunches to burn belly fat. You can do all sorts of exercises, such as:

- Weight bearing exercises will increase muscle mass all over your body and end up burning more calories and will use your abdominals to stabilize yourself during the workout.

- Get your cardio going to help you burn extra calories and get rid of excess fat. Walking, running and jogging provide overall fitness and will keep your weight in check. Try to make your heart pound every day for at least twenty minutes.

- Keeping great posture is a great way to help you get your flat stomach. When you stand up tall your abdomen instantly looks flatter. Suck in or hold in your tummy, put your shoulders back and lift your rib cage, and voila, you have a flatter stomach instantly!

- Practicing Pilates is an outstanding way to improve core strength and get flatter abdominals. Pilates will help to keep that muscle memory of how to hold good posture as well. You abdominal muscles are part of a network of muscles called your core, and they are responsible for supporting and holding your body safely.

- Do exercises that strengthen your core and improve your posture. Push-ups, planks and hovers (elbow plank) are amazing target exercises. These types of exercises will strengthen your core and flatten you abdomen. They also tone up your entire body and build lean muscles mass.

- Yoga is another great way to encourage breathing and stress relief. Breathing slowly and relaxing will help you with belly fat.

- If you reach a plateau or get tired of your routine, shake it up. Change up what types of recreation and fitness you are doing to inspire change and enthusiasm. There are many challenges available online and many resources for abdominal workouts. Most important, have fun when your exercise!

- Eat healthy and regularly- Contrary to popular belief, starving yourself will not help you lose belly fat. Cutting your caloric intake, on the other hand, will (particularly cutting out empty calories). If you skip meals you are promoting a slow metabolism and low energy. An effective strategy is to switch to five smaller lighter meals per day (rather than having three large meals) as smaller portions more often will leave you feeling less hungry and keep energy levels up on a more consistent basis throughout the day. Wait twenty minutes after eating, as it takes that amount of time for your body to realize it has eaten enough. This is also beneficial for digestion.

- As always, eat whole, healthy, nutritious foods. As you've learned, foods high in sugar, artificial chemicals and those that are highly processed, do not benefit your health or your weight management goals. Be sure to look at labels when you purchase your food. Even food for weight-loss can be full of sodium and chemicals. In particular, avoid foods with high sodium content as excessive consumption of salt makes the body retain water and this makes the abdomen appear bloated. Avoid foods that have white or artificial sugars in them. Instead, choose foods such as fresh berries, yogurt, or natural sugars, like maple syrup or unpasturized honey to help with your cravings. Be sure to make your own meals as often as you can, that way you control what you put into your body and your portion size. Finally, be sure to avoid false claims and supplement promises. The only way to a flat abdomen is to eat clean and exercise.

- Keep trying to reach your goal- Stay focused and keep going; you will get there! With dedication and devotion you will reach your goal. Make sure that you keep your goal present in your conscious thinking often. Perhaps you can put a photo of the stomach you desire right on the fridge or the cookie pantry. Have a specific goal in mind for your weight-loss. It is important to have a realistic goal and keep it in mind with a timeline and action plan. This goal will help you stay motivated on the days you don't feel like going to the gym and staying on track. Get plenty of sleep and avoid alcohol in excess. Avoid stress in your life. It might be surprising, but as mentioned earlier in the stress section of the book, stress can cause weight-gain and belly fat. Remember to hold yourself accountable and stay motivated by keeping a food journal, joining a group exercise class with a friend and reward yourself for small accomplishments. We're almost there!

- Improve your digestion: Unzip your jeans after a meal and let your bloated belly out. Don't feel bad, many people have issues with bloating after eating and the problem can be easily solved. Be sure to rule out any medical condition by checking with your Doctor first. But you can improve your digestion to prevent that bloat after meals. We discussed many of these tips in great detail in the beginning of the program. Here is a reminder list of suggestions. Calm down when your eat so you are in a relaxed response and not stressed. Chew your food thoroughly to help break down the food, maintain good posture so your stomach isn't compressed, decrease hard to digest dairy, eat smaller meals, be mindful while eating, sit down to eat, sip on ginger tea, eat largest meal at lunch, avoid late night eating, eat good quality, nutrient dense foods, breathe while you eat, take your time to eat, slow down and give yourself time to eat and enjoy.

- Try an abdominal challenge workout: There are so many abdominal challenges available to you on the internet and around the gym. Find a reputable source or seek out a personal trainer to create one for you or you can create a challenge for yourself. I suggest you find a workout that excites you. My favourite lately, are 30 day abdominal challenges. I like sticking to it for a month. Usually I put a plan into a calendar, and try to follow it for a month. It is super motivating and fun to try. The results are amazing!

- Try Pilates - The Pilates technique, designed by Joseph Pilates, is a great workout for your core. It is designed to integrate your entire body all while challenging your core. Since Pilates strengthens your entire abdominal region and encourages a holding in contraction, you will gain muscle memory to hold your belly in and flat. Pilates isn't just crunches, it is so much more. It trains your body to be able to hold itself in proper alignment. Not only will you gain the ability to hold your belly in and flat, it will help to improve your posture as well.

*Be the best version of yourself...*

*"There are ways to cut cravings by naturally balancing your blood sugar."*

— *Mark Hyman*

# — WEEK NINE —

## Nutrition Management

By keeping your blood sugar levels under control, you
can lose fat, regulate mood, and boost energy levels.
Eating a lot of fiber can help you to lose weight and
regulate blood sugar levels.

**Blood sugar level regulation is important for
you along your Mission:**

You are full of energy one minute and fatigued and grumpy the
next. Why? Your blood sugar levels are all out of balance. Blood sugar
plays an important role in many of our bodily functions, including
energy and mood, and can also greatly affect your weight management efforts. The body strives to maintain blood sugar levels within
a narrow range through the coordinated effort of several glands and

their hormones. If these mechanisms are disrupted, diabetes (high blood sugar), hypoglycemia (low blood sugar), and weight gain may result. Ideally your blood sugar levels gradually rise when you eat and gently fall as the sugar is absorbed into your cells. When you live an unhealthy lifestyle, such as lack of exercise and poor diet, you disrupt this gentle cycle.

Your blood sugar levels can negatively affect you regardless of your health condition. You don't have to be diabetic to feel and notice the negative effects that low and/or high blood sugar levels play on mood and energy levels. Whether you're looking to get better control over your blood sugar levels to increase energy, improve your mood, or prevent health problems and weight gain, the following information will help you obtain a better understanding of the role food has on your health and your ability to manage your weight.

### Blood sugar levels and the link between diabetes, hypoglycemia, and weight gain:

While regulating blood sugar levels is crucial to weight loss it is also essential to mood regulation and prevention of serious health problems such as diabetes and hypoglycemia. Blood sugar problems are strongly correlated with the so-called 'western diet'. This diet is rich in refined sugar, fat and animal products, and low in dietary fiber. It is widely accepted that refined carbohydrates and sugar are the most important contributing factors to diabetes and re-active hypoglycemia, obesity and mood disturbances. Refined sugars are quickly absorbed into the blood stream, causing a rapid increase in blood sugar. The body responds by dumping a large amount of insulin from the pancreas. Insulin acts as a key to your cell door to dump sugar into the cells. The excessive secretion of insulin drives blood sugar levels down, often so low that it results in symptoms associated with hypoglycemia.

In response to the rapid drop, the adrenal glands try to compensate and secrete the stress hormone, epinephrine (adrenaline). With the presence of epinephrine, stored glycogen from the liver rapidly enters back into your blood stream. Blood sugar levels tend to rise and fall numerous times in response to refined and processed foods. In time, the adrenal glands become exhausted by the repeated stress and cannot mount an appropriate response. This lack of response leads to hypoglycemia or low blood sugar. When blood sugar levels are low, you don't feel good, your energy levels are low and your ability to deal with stress decreases. When blood sugar levels drop, we crave more sugar or refined carbohydrates to bring blood levels back up. Moreover, the stress the body underwent when blood sugar levels were low caused a cortisol (a stress hormone) increase. As your body deals with this drastic rise and drop in glucose levels, you end up producing excess insulin. This results in excess glucose in the cells, which ends up being converted and stored as fat. If all of these control mechanisms are further stressed, the body will eventually become insensitive to insulin, the pancreas will become exhausted, and hypoglycemia will turn into diabetes (high blood sugar levels). The by-product is weight gain and instability in mood.

The good news is that keeping blood sugar levels under control can help you stay healthy, regulate mood and prevent weight gain. The most critical component of managing diabetes, hypoglycemia, weight gain, and mood fluctuations, is regulating blood sugar levels through natural nutrition. You can avoid these abrupt swings in blood sugar levels by choosing natural foods that are ingested with full fiber and natural nutrients. When food is in its natural state the body knows how much insulin to properly secrete and the rate of absorption into the body is slower, thus the body has gentle rises and gentle falls in the blood sugar levels.

*The key to mood regulation, weight management, and decreased fat storage is to keep the blood sugar levels steady.*

### The glycemic index can be your tool to manage blood sugar levels:

The glycemic index was founded by Dr. David Jenkins, a Canadian professor at the University of Toronto, and a world leader in nutrition research. Originally established to help improve blood sugar control in patients with diabetes, it has since paved the way for many of today's popular diets! The glycemic index classifies carbohydrate-containing foods according to their potential to raise your blood sugar level. Food is scored between 0-100 and usually uses glucose as a reference. The index is a strong tool that measures if food raises blood sugar levels dramatically, moderately or a just little bit. Carbohydrate-containing foods that break down slowly, releasing glucose gradually into the blood stream, have low GI values. Carbohydrate-containing foods that break down quickly during digestion are highest on the index because their response is fast and high. The GI index has become an important tool for helping us select the right foods to help stabilize our blood sugar levels.

### Foods ranked by Jenkins glycemic index are given scores:

- High: 70 and up. Examples include instant white rice, brown rice, plain white bread, white skinless baked potato, boiled red potatoes with skin and watermelon.
- Medium: 56 to 69. Examples include sweet corn, bananas, raw

pineapple, raisins and certain types of ice cream.
- Low: 55 and under. Examples include raw carrots, peanuts, raw apple, grapefruit, peas, skim milk, kidney beans and lentils.

### How does the GI index help with weight management?

For many years, I have been educating my clients on the effects foods play on blood sugar levels because the approach to weight-loss is about over-all health and sustainability. And, understanding this relationship among blood-sugar imbalances, food and health is a very powerful motivating factor in the weight-loss journey. The theory behind diets based on the glycemic index is that foods with a low GI value slowly release sugar into the blood, providing you with a steady supply of energy, leaving you feeling satisfied longer so that you're less likely to snack. In contrast, foods with a high GI value cause a rapid, but short-lived rise in blood sugar. This leaves you lacking in energy and feeling hungry within a short time, with the result that you end up reaching for a snack. If this pattern is frequently repeated, you're likely to gain weight as a result of constantly overeating.

### Benefits of using the glycemic index:
- Will fill you up, keep you satisfied for longer, and help you burn more of your body fat and less of your body muscle
- Will enable you to increase your food intake without increasing your waistline
- Will assist you in controlling your appetite
- Will regulate your mood because of the stabilizing of blood sugar levels; these foods will support the functions of the body

## Not all carbohydrates are created equal:

So, following a strict GI diet, for example, is not recommended here. There are some important factors that influence the way carbohydrates are metabolized and therefore influence your blood-sugar levels. The overall nutrient content of a food will affect its GI. For example, fat and protein affect the absorption of carbohydrates. How you cook a food, the degree of processing, and the ripeness and variety of a fruit, for example, also affect its GI. Even the structure of the carbohydrate itself influences the GI. For example, processed instant oatmeal has a higher GI than traditional rolled oats used to make porridge. This is because, as a result of processing, the starch in instant oats is more easily exposed to digestive enzymes, causing it to break down and enter the bloodstream more rapidly. Meanwhile, some foods have low GI values because they are packed with fibre, which acts as a physical barrier slowing down the absorption of carbohydrates into the blood. GI index charts, therefore, only identify the effect different foods have on blood sugar levels when they are eaten on their own, and consequently, many nutritionists believe this is one of the main problems with GI diets. When you eat a mixture of foods together in a meal, the GI value of that whole meal will change. As a guideline though, the more low GI foods you include in a meal, the lower the overall GI value of that meal will be. In general, most nutritionists and dietitians are supportive of the basic principles of the GI diet. They do, however, believe that you shouldn't get too hung up about avoiding all high GI foods because when foods are eaten together in a meal, that meal can have a very different GI value to the individual foods it contains.

## Various Carbohydrates:

Carbohydrates are your body's primary source of fuel. The body breaks carbohydrates down to glucose, your body's preferred energy source. Most sugars are digested, absorbed and converted to glucose, some glucose cannot be digested and this is in the form of fiber. Different carbohydrates will produce different effects on blood sugar levels.

**Complex carbohydrates-** Complex carbohydrates, or starch, are simply sugars bonded together to form a chain. It is more complex so to speak, the more bonds the more complex and longer it takes to break down the carboydrate. Digestive enzymes have to work much harder to access the bonds to break the chain into individual sugars for absorption through the intestines. For this reason, digestion of complex carbohydrates takes longer. The slow absorption of sugars provides us with a steady supply of energy and limits the amount of sugar converted into fat! Due to refining and processing many of the complex carbohydrates are not as complex as they are naturally and this disrupts the absorption time. The 'new' carbohydrate creates an inappropriate insulin response by your body and too much insulin is secreted. The blood sugar levels rise quicker due to the simpler bonds and lack of fiber resulting in an increase in insulin secretion. The excess insulin makes the blood sugar levels drop off quickly and also allows for glucose and insulin to be stored as fat. When you choose foods that are as close to their natural state as possible you will eliminate the preceding scenario from happening.

**Simple carbohydrates-** Simple carbohydrates are smaller molecules of sugar, unlike the long chains in starch. For example, the individual sugars - fructose, and galactose (monosaccharides), or two sugars bonded together (disaccharides), are small simple carbohydrates. They are digested quickly because the individual sugars are ready to be absorbed immediately, plus digestive enzymes have easy access to the bonds in the paired molecules. You could say most of the work has been done! Their rapid absorption increases the chance of sugar being converted to fat but only if there is an abundance of energy absorbed. Because your cells usually do not require that amount of energy at one time, they are full. The sugar must either be converted to glycogen (sugar storage in cells) or converted to fat. The cell can only store a limited amount of glycogen so in many cases simple carbohydrates may contribute to fat stores. This rule can change if the glycogen levels are low such as after exercise. Other natural foods like fruit, honey and maple syrup contain naturally occurring simple sugars, however because the amount of energy is lower and they contain natural fiber there is less chance for sugar to be converted to fat. Plus many fruits are high in fiber which helps slow digestion, again limiting the flood of sugar into cells when it's not needed!

## Why are carbohydrates important?

Carbohydrates are the body's primary source of clean burning fuel. The energy can be released quickly and easily to fulfill any immediate requirements within cells. Carbohydrates do not require oxygen to burn therefore they fuel most muscular contractions, meaning our carbohydrate intake is very important for regular exercise sessions. If carbohydrate stores are low, exercise and movement will seem like a big effort! Refined and processed (simple and complex) carbohydrates, like sugar and bread, highly elevate the blood sugar. Unrefined natural simple and complex carbohydrates, like fruit and vegetables, do not affect blood sugar levels substantially. These foods enter the body with nutritional value and natural fiber, all of which sustain blood sugar levels.

## The value of fiber:

Want to lose weight? Eat foods high in fiber. Add this secret weapon to your eating plan. Filling your meals with high fiber foods will keep your calorie count low, help regulate blood sugar levels and help you lose weight too. A diet high in fiber can also help you control certain medical conditions by helping you control your weight, but fiber can also benefit you as it travels through your digestive system. It helps to regulate the rate of absorption of your food into your body, thereby regulating blood sugar levels. Fiber also makes you feel full and satisfied and keeps your bowels functioning well. Fiber is the part of whole grains, vegetables, fruits, and nuts that resists digestion in the stomach and intestines. Dietary fiber offers many health benefits from weight management to cardiovascular health. However, the Canadian Diabetes Association report fiber consumption is at an all time low average. Fiber can help to regulate blood sugar levels, help with weight loss, and is good for your overall health. It is time to start roughing it, Literally!

## What is fiber?

Fiber is one of those nutrients that many of us know is important but are not necessarily clear on exactly what it is. Basically, the term fiber refers to carbohydrates that cannot be digested. Sounds like it is not important then, right? Wrong. Fiber is present in all plants that are eaten for food, including fruits, vegetables, grains and legumes. Not all fiber is the same though, there are a couple ways it is categorized.

Usually it is categorized by how it absorbs water. Soluble fiber partially absorbs water. Insoluble fiber does not absorb in water. Bottom line fiber is an important part of a healthy lifestyle. Most fiber is made up of many glucose molecules and does not break down into glucose before it goes to the colon, and often not even in the colon is it broken down.

Even so, fiber does have a great effect on our digestion along the way. Fiber is bulky so it tends to make us feel full. Fiber holds onto water and creates a sense of feeling full. The content of the stomach more gradually leaves due to fiber, thereby regulating absorption and blood sugar levels. The presence of insoluble fiber tends to speed up the transit time through the small intestines and the gel like soluble fiber slows things down. In the colon, fiber absorbs excess water waste and toxins and creates bulk to keep things moving. As you can see both soluble and insoluble fiber types are important in your diet. Soluble fiber attracts fluid in your digestive tract and forms a slow-moving thick sludge. This slows digestion to give time for nutrients to be absorbed. Insoluble fiber stays intact and sweeps through the digestive tract pushing or sweeping waste through. This type of fiber also helps create bulk and movement to pass bowels easier.

**Sources of Insoluble fiber:** Insoluble fiber is the tough hard to chew parts of grain and produce. Salads with lots of veggies include a lot of insoluble fiber. Some  more examples of foods containing insoluble fiber are; Cabbage, lettuce, kale, onions, peppers, carrots, cucumbers, grapes and popcorn. Dried fruits, including prunes, dates and apricots are a well known insoluble fiber great for the bowl function.

**Sources of soluble fiber:** Soluble fiber is the softer easier part of grain and produce. Whole grains, rice oatmeal are chock full of insoluble fiber. Some vegetables and fruit and legumes contain soluble fiber as well. When water is added to food the soluble fiber thickens. Soluble fiber acts as the absorber. It absorbs water.

### The role fiber plays on your blood sugar levels:

Fiber offers many benefits in the prevention, control and treatment of blood sugar issues. Diabetes is characterized by sustained high blood sugar levels and hypoglycemia is characterized by sustain low blood sugar levels. It tends to develop when the body isn't regulating insulin levels properly. Fiber is capable of slowing down the absorption of carbohydrates, thereby preventing rapid rises and thus falls in blood sugar levels. Fiber increases the sensitivity of tissues to insulin, thereby preventing the excessive secretion of insulin; fiber also improves the uptake of glucose by the liver and other tissues, thereby preventing a sustained elevation of blood sugar. Due to the regulatory effect fiber has on blood sugar levels it is also good for weight management, mood regulation and diabetes. Fiber prevents excess insulin secretion and decreases fat storage. Fiber is also great for feeling full and leads to consumption of fewer calories. Fewer calories results in weight-loss.

### How fiber helps with weight-loss:

The great news is that fiber alone contains no calories. It provides the bulk of your diet that gives you the satisfaction of chewing, plus the feeling of being full. Fiber prevents excess insulin secretion and decreases fat storage. Less fat storage is great for managing your weight. Fiber is also great for feeling full and leads to consumption of fewer calories. Fewer calories results in weight-loss. Insoluble fiber, found in vegetables and whole grain breads and cereals, adds bulk to the diet and does not easily absorb water. Soluble fiber, found in fruits, legumes, seeds, and oat products, exits the stomach more slowly and helps your stomach feel full for a longer period of time. Fiber has other benefits that can help you on your Mission. For example, foods containing fiber take longer to eat, which equates to eating slower, your stomach feels more full, so you ultimately eat less. Food that has more fiber is also more satisfying so you don't feel as hungry between meals. You eat less when you feel full. Foods high in fiber also enter the blood stream slower so you experience more regulated blood sugar levels and energy levels. Fiber also acts like a sponge in your digestive tract, absorbing other molecules  and the calories that they have as carbs, sugar, and fat. Bottom line, fiber makes you feel full and satisfied longer and leads to a more accurate evaluation of what your body needs, preventing over eating. It also brings you sustained energy, energy you can use to burn calories.

### How can fiber affect your health?

A diet high in fiber and the usual weight loss that is associated with an increase in fiber can reduce your risk of many medical conditions. You already know that fiber helps with weight management, digestion and blood sugar regulation, but did you know it can have big benefits on you heart health, skin health, and over all well being.

### What are the best sources of fiber?

Eat a variety of high-fiber foods to receive the benefits from both the insoluble foods and the soluble foods, including raw vegetables and fruits with the skins. In addition, drink plenty of fluids. Eight glasses of liquid are recommended a day because fibrous foods draw water from the intestines so you will require more water. When you select unprocessed, unrefined options that are as close to their natural state as possible, you will be getting the natural amount of fiber your body needs.  Shop for good, nutritional food and you will add this important part of fiber to your diet.

- Shop for fresh produce twice a week. Many vegetables lose their nutrients during prolonged refrigeration.
- Eat whole fruits instead of fruit juices.
- Avoid wilted vegetables and bruised fruits.
- Replace white or whole-wheat rice, breads and cereals with brown and whole grain products.
- For breakfast, choose the cereals that have whole grain as the first ingredient and avoid sugar.
- Choose small, young vegetables.
- Snack on raw vegetables.
- Select whole grain products for more fiber instead of "enriched" breads or refined pastas.
- Substitute beans or legumes for some of your meat planned meals.
- Visit larger stores or health food stores for whole-grain flours and hard-to-find nuts and seeds.

**More tips to help manage blood sugar levels and increase fiber:**

A diet high in complex carbohydrates and dietary fiber, and low in fat is clearly the diet of choice to regulate blood sugar levels and manage weight. Here are some more specific dietary guidelines for good food selections.

**Vegetables** Vegetables provide the broadest range of nutrients of any food class. They are rich sources of vitamins, minerals, carbohydrates, and protein. The little fat they contain is in the form of essential fatty acids. Vegetables provide valuable health promoting benefits with fiber; it therefore keeps blood sugar levels in check. There are a couple of vegetables to watch out for, which are higher on the glycemic index. They include: potatoes, yams, squash, and corn, and should be eaten in moderation. Include garlic and onions in your meals as they can significantly regulate blood sugar level and help improve insulin productivity.

**Fruit:** Fruits are a rich source of many beneficial compounds. Regular fruit consumption has been shown to offer significant protection against many chronic degenerative diseases, among them cancer, heart disease, cataracts, strokes and complication with diabetes. Although a simple carbohydrate, the blood stream absorbs fructose (fruit sugar) slowly, thereby allowing the body time to utilize it. Fruits are also an excellent source of vitamins and minerals as well as health promoting fiber compounds.

**Whole grain breads, cereals, and pastas:** These are considered to be complex carbohydrates and enter the blood stream slowly, providing they are not processed. Once carbohydrates are processed and refined, they are like simple sugars and cause a significant rise in the blood sugar levels. Choose whole grain products like, brown rice, bulgur, kasha, kamut, spelt, quinoa and rye. Choose rye, spelt or nut breads over brown or white wheat breads, bagels and buns. Choose kamut, spelt or rice pasta over white or whole wheat pasta. Choose ancient grain cereals like spelt, kamut, and quinoa instead of commercial brand cereals. Choose real oats sweetened with maple syrup instead of the instant oatmeal cereals with sugar. Choose rice, spelt or rye crackers instead of whole wheat and white flour crackers. Make a habit of buying nothing but unprocessed and unrefined foods for better blood sugar regulation and keep your energy levels high.

**Legumes** Legumes are fantastic foods. They are rich in important nutrients and health promoting compounds. Legumes help improve liver function and they lower cholesterol. They are extremely effective in improving blood sugar control. They also provide an amazing amount of fiber and are extremely important in weight-loss plans and in the dietary management of diabetes. Legumes can be combined with whole grains like brown rice to form what is known as a complete protein. Example of legumes include: chick peas, black beans, kidney beans.

**Fats and oils:** Saturated fats are known to have a negative effect on glucose control and they are linked to both diabetes and hypoglycemia. Avoiding margarine, deep-fried foods and rancid oils is a great idea to improve your general health. Good quality fats and oils called essential fatty acids (EFA's) found in nuts and seeds, fish, eggs and flax seed oils, are required by the body for nerve function, cellular function, communication pathways, blood pressure regulation, and control of inflammation just to name a few. Good quality fats also regulate the absorption and utilization of carbohydrates.

### Other suggestions

- B vitamins help stimulate insulin secretion and regulate blood sugar levels as well as produce energy.
- Take a multi-vitamin with chromium or glucose tolerance factor to help you regulate blood sugar levels.

- Keep normal sleeping and eating habits.

- Avoid stressful situations.

- Oatmeal contains a significant amount of B vitamins, chromium, and fiber that are beneficial for managing blood sugar levels.

- Moderate exercise, including breathing exercises and fresh air, are good ideas.

- Drink plenty of water.

- Eat at regular intervals; never go three hours without eating to prevent drops in blood sugar levels.

Regulating your blood sugar levels is one of the most effective ways to manage your weight. Keep blood sugar levels regulated; watch your energy soar, your mood stabilize and the pounds melt away. Controlling your weight is more manageable with fiber and a nutritious diet. Fiber will not solve all your weight control problems, but it is a step in the right direction. A regular daily intake of fiber will help you regulate your blood sugar levels and will help you maintain and manage weight - even if you are healthy and at your ideal weight. By monitoring and managing your blood sugar levels through low GI foods, healthy carbohydrates, and fiber you will be much more successful at losing, managing and maintaining weight for the rest of your life!

This week allow yourself to find happiness and acceptance while on your Mission. Use the tools and the benefits of managing your expectations to help find a good balance between expectations and acceptance. Take a 30-day challenge to lose belly fat for a flatter stomach. Stay motivated and feel fantastic. Keep your blood sugar levels under control, and watch how you can lose fat, regulate mood, and boost your energy levels. Try to increase the amount of fiber you consume, as it can help you to lose weight and regulate blood sugar levels. Remember: There are two ways to be happy: Improve your reality or lower your expectations; lowering your expectations simply is not an option for us, when you have selected Mission Slim Possible! I often say in my classes near the end of a tough workout, "Yes you can" and yes you can!

# STAY ON TARGET

## MY WEEKLY CHECKLIST

- ☑ Find things to be happy about
- ☑ Manage your expectations
- ☑ Take 30-day challenge
- ☑ Regulate blood sugar levels
- ☑ Increase fiber rich foods
- ☑ Improve your reality
- ☐ _____
- ☐ _____
- ☐ _____
- ☐ _____
- ☐ _____
- ☐ _____
- ☐ _____
- ☐ _____
- ☐ _____
- ☐ _____
- ☐ _____

## MY WEIGHT THIS WEEK:

Began at:_____

Finished at:_____

Total weight loss:_____

## MY MEASUREMENTS THIS WEEK:

### BEGAN AT

Shoulders:_____

Chest:_____

Waist:_____

Hips:_____

### FINISHED AT

Shoulders:_____

Chest:_____

Waist:_____

Hips:_____

### DIFFERENCE/TOTAL INCHES LOST:

Shoulders:_____

Chest:_____

Waist:_____

Hips:_____

What really resonated for me this week?

_____
_____
_____
_____
_____
_____
_____
_____
_____
_____

What worked well for me this week?

_____
_____
_____
_____
_____
_____
_____
_____
_____
_____
_____

# WEEK TEN

## Psychology Management/Self-Coaching

Self-hypnosis and using the power of your mind can help you on your Mission. Program your mind for success!

## Recreation Management

Adopt a lifestyle of active living and recreation. Permanent weight management is a lifestyle.

## Nutrition Management

Ayurveda can be your natural path to a slim and happy life.

*"The mind is powerful, and you have more control than you think."*

*— Scott.D Lewis*

# — WEEK TEN —

## Psychology Management/Self- Coaching

Self-hypnosis and using the power of your mind can help you on your Mission. Program your mind for success!

**Self-hypnosis and using the power of your mind can help you on your Mission:**

Have you ever wondered how people become hypnotized? Do you sometimes wonder if you have to be suggestive in order for it to happen? Everyone can become hypnotized, here's how to use Hypnosis or the power of your mind to your advantage for your Mission. Self-hypnosis and guided meditation are very similar concepts and have similar results. To understand hypnosis or the power of suggestion, you need to appreciate the nature of suggestion and how it works.

## What is self-hypnosis?

Hypnosis, also referred to as hypnotherapy or self-hypnosis, is a totally safe, yet powerful tool that can help you gain control over unwanted behaviors, habits, emotions and thoughts. In essence, therapeutic hypnosis is a relaxed, natural, yet focused, state of mind that allows you to become mentally open to receiving positive suggestions and images. Hypnosis is very similar if not the same as guided mediation and the use of affirmation in a relaxed state. Hypnosis is so natural that you routinely enter and exit hypnotic trances several times a day, such as while driving or while watching TV! Hypnosis is a state of mind ideal for learning quickly for making changes in an instant. The hypnotic process is a natural process, and it is a choice to allow yourself the pleasure of connecting inside yourself. Hypnosis, like meditation, is a useful tool for achieving deep relaxation. Self-hypnosis is when you hypnotize or meditate yourself. This is often more practical as a stress management tool than normal hypnosis, as you do not need to have a hypnotist present. Drawing on the same "relaxation response" that drives meditation, self-hypnosis helps you to relax your body, lets stress hormones subside, and calms your mind. The relaxation achieved with self-hypnosis is much like the relaxation experienced during meditation. Self-hypnosis is like mixing meditation and affirmations, we often use affirmations as part of self-hypnosis to manage stress and build self-confidence. Affirmations are the positive statements that we make to ourselves. Along with meditation and imagery, self-hypnosis can usefully be used along your Mission. This deep hypnosis is often compared to the relaxed mental state between wakefulness and sleep. We often go into relaxed, hypnotic states during the day. Hypnosis can be used to relax and calm the mind and become concentrated and peaceful, while adding suggestions into the subconscious mind.

## How does self-hypnosis or meditative affirmations work?

Positive thoughts breed positive action, which bring about positive changes. That's exactly how hypnosis works. Hypnosis or 'meditative affirmations', if you will, help install new feelings of well-being and reprogram your mind positively. Since hypnosis is accessing the creative unconscious part of the mind, there is a greater ability to accept positive suggestions. Meditative affirmations can often be much more effective, and produce much quicker results, than with doing affirmations in an awake alert state. It is a relaxed state characterized by extreme suggestibility, relaxation and heightened imagination. It's not really like sleep, because you are alert the whole time. It is most often compared to daydreaming or meditating. You are fully aware, but you tune out most of the sounds and stimuli from around you. The school of thought on hypnosis is that it is a method to access your subconscious mind more directly. Normally, we are most aware of the thought processes that occur in our conscious awake mind. You consciously think over new things you are learning, consciously choose words as you speak, consciously try to remember where you left your wallet. But when you do these things, your conscious mind is working hand-in-hand with your subconscious mind, the unconscious part of your mind that does your "behind the scenes" thinking. Your subconscious mind has access to a vast amount of information that lets you solve problems, create sentences or locate your wallet. It puts plans and ideas together and helps run your conscious mind.

Your subconscious takes care of all the stuff you do automatically. Why is this important? You don't actively work through the steps of walking minute to minute -- your subconscious mind does that. You don't think through every little thing you do while driving a car. Your subconscious mind is actually in charge of much of your behaviour. In reality, your subconscious mind is the real brains behind your operation because it does most of your thinking, and it decides a lot of what you do. You can see how important it is to have your subconscious mind programed well. When you're awake, your conscious mind works to take in and absorb your world, make decisions and put behaviour into action. It also takes in new information and relays it to the subconscious mind.

Deep relaxation and focusing exercises such as affirmation, meditation and hypnosis, work to calm the busy conscious mind so that it can step back and take a break from the role in your thinking process. In this state, you're still aware of what's going on, but your awake conscious mind can take a backseat to your subconscious portion of your mind. Effectively, this allows you to be in direct contact with the subconscious.

### How does hypnosis help in relation to weight-loss?

Weight-loss hypnosis may help you shed extra pounds when it's part of applying all the tips along your Mission Slim Possible. Hypnosis is a state of inner absorption and concentration, like being relaxed. When you're meditating with affirmations or trying self-hypnosis, your attention is highly focused, and you're more open to suggestions, including behavior changes that can help you lose weight. IT is one of many tools you can use to help stay focused on your Mission.

**Getting started with self-hypnosis and meditative affirmations:**

With the proper relaxation and focusing techniques, almost everyone can enter a hypnotic relaxed meditative state for themselves and make their own suggestions to the unconscious mind. Self-hypnosis is useful for boosting your confidence, encouraging yourself towards a healthier lifestyle and improving your performance. It is a great tool to use to help get you closer to your target. Follow these basic steps to help you move towards your desired goals:

1. Think about what you would like to achieve or change, state your goal in a single sentence and remember what it is you want to focus on for yourself.

2. Choose a relaxing quiet place in which you are completely comfortable and prepare the space to limit distractions.

3. Play relaxing music, light a candle, or burn incense to help you relax deeply. Remove any distractions.

4. Close your eyes and take a few deep breaths. Progressively relax your entire body from head to toe. Talk yourself through relaxing each body part.

5. Count down from ten to one and tell yourself that with each number you'll become more and more relaxed, perfectly at peace, perfectly relaxed, both physically and mentally, and go deeper into relaxation.

6. When you're in a deeply relaxed state, start using your goal statement, and make it as vivid as possible in your imagination.

Then simply let go. Go with it and notice everything about what is great about your desired goal. trust that you have handed it over to your unconscious mind, and that you are training your subconscious mind. Spend some time here. Hold the image as long and vivid as possible. Use your affirmations here as well. Your positive statements will help you get to your target.

7. Count yourself awake, up from one to ten, and tell yourself that you're wide awake, ready for the day, fresh and alert. Feel thrilled your unconscious mind is now helping you reach your goals.

*No one will do it for you....*
*you got this*

**It's time for self-coaching and inner reflection:**

Take time to answer and work through these questions in your journal to help keep you focused and on a clear path towards your goals. By taking action you will bring your goals into your life. These self-coaching questions will help clarify what you need to have accomplished this week.

## Self-Coaching Questions

- What needs to happen each day this week?
- What are my priorities this week?
- How will these action steps help me get closer to my goals?
- In the next week my complete focus will be on?
- My direction is clear to me because...?
- I am willing to commit to...?
- What might success look like to me for this week?
- What resonated and stood out to me from the program and what impact will it have on me this week?
- I deserve this because...?
- I am thrilled with myself because...?
- Why is it important for me to take action and follow my goals this week?

# — NOTES —

"A vigorous five mile walk will do more good for an unhappy but otherwise healthy adult than all the medicine and psychology in the world".

— Paul Dudley

# — WEEK TEN —

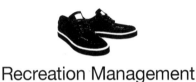

## Recreation Management

A life long commitment to active living and
being recreational!

### What is active living?

You hear a lot about living a healthy lifestyle, enough that the phrase 'healthy lifestyle' has become mainstream. The problem is, that phrase describes the life we need to live if we want to feel good and look good. Committing to staying fit and being active can be a challenge, but the rewards out number the drawbacks of not being active. So, what does active living actually mean? Eating habits have a direct impact on our health and an active lifestyle along with a healthy diet is undoubtably important for over all physical fitness and well-being. Being physically active provides you with numerous benefits.

Active living includes everyday activities such as, walking, dancing, housework, gardening, cycling, swimming, cross-country skiing, golfing, and many other activities. Physical activity is an important part of a healthy active lifestyle. With the development of technology, the modern lifestyle has become very sedentary. The moment you stop being active, the benefits also start to stop. The excessive use of: computers, gadgets, elevators, escalators, and cars have substantially decreased most of our physical activities. It is therefore very important to instill some discipline into our lives for our own well being by maintaining not only sound eating habits, but also an active lifestyle that involves lots of physical activities. Exercising is easier than we think and it is not necessary to hit the gym everyday to stay in shape and be active. An early morning jog or brisk walk followed by some simple workouts or little bit of Yoga can go a long way in keeping you fit, active and healthy. Skipping rope and biking can also be a fun and healthy way to get some good physical exercise.

Active living is a way of life in which people are physically active during their day. It means walking or bicycling often and maybe even to work. It means walking to pick the kids up from school. It also means exercising or playing in the park, taking the stairs and going to recreation fun facilities. It means signing up for the tennis league. For children, active living includes participating in physical classes and being active during recess at school. Daily physical activity is important, we have to work it into our day-to-day activities in order to be consistent with it. As mentioned in week one of the program, Walking is one of the best ways to keep active. Even walking just a little bit helps. It allows you to live a healthier life, as well as a better quality of life.

By deciding to keep active you promote a healthy, well functioning machine that is your body. Active living is an approach to life that values and includes physical activity in everyday living. You can find ways to be active at school, at home, at work and during leisure time, at any time of the year. Physical exercise is any type of physical exertion or activity performed to develop or maintain physical fitness and overall health. The Ministry of Health Promotion, recommends that adults over the age of 18 need to be physically active 30-60 minutes, most days of the week, to stay healthy. The actual time you spend depends on the intensity and degree of effort. There is mounting evidence that exercising can be done either in one session, or it can also be broken down into multiple shorter sessions without losing any of the wonderful benefits. Physical activity doesn't need to be hard or intense. The effort you expend, even if you are just starting out, will be beneficial. Even just a few minutes a day can improve your health and overall feelings of well-being. Remember every little bit of effort contributes.

## Why is active living important?

There are many benefits to being physically active and living an active fit life. Benefits from regular physical activity include, better physical and mental health, more energy, better circulation from movement, weight management or loss, stronger muscles and bones, stronger immune system and reduced stress. Numerous studies and research confirm the important role that physical activity can play in the prevention of, or reducing the occurrence of, many diseases and illnesses, such as heart disease, obesity, high blood pressure, Type II diabetes, osteoporosis, stroke, depression, colon and breast cancer, etc. It's never too late to get started – a little walk every day can help a long the way to reduce your risk of illness and weight gain. Perhaps people put off exercise and active living because they think it must be difficult or time-consuming in order to be beneficial. In fact, you don't have to train like an intense tri-athlete to reap the benefits. According to Canada's Physical Activity Guide to Healthy Living (a companion guide to Canada's Food Guide to Healthy Eating), you will gain significant health benefits just by adding physical activity to your daily routine. Your benefits will increase as you add more activities to your day. That is pretty amazing, that just by increasing your activity, you also increase the benefits. The more you are active the more benefits you will experience. Exercise does more for you than just help you lose weight. Regular physical activity is a prescription from many doctors for helping decrease stress; relieve depression, anxiety, heartburn and constipation; increase happiness; improve your love life and fitness level; and help prevent diabetes, heart disease, weight gain, osteoporosis and cancer. Being active is a key factor, therefore, in the health and quality of life for all ages. It is essential for healthy growth and development in our children: it develops a strong, healthy heart; muscular strength and flexibility, and bone density. It also contributes to building positive self-esteem, and setting healthy habits for life.

**According to Ontario Ministry of Health and Long-term Care, regular physical activity provides almost limitless benefits, including:**

1 Maintenance of healthy weight.

2 Reduced stress levels.

3 Relieved symptoms of depression and anxiety.

4 Increased energy.

5 Improved sleep and digestion.

6   Improved posture and balance.

7   Stronger muscles and bones.

8   More confidence and a more positive outlook on life.

9   Ability to perform daily tasks with more ease and less fatigue.

10   Increased bone density.

11   Better circulation.

12   Strengthened heart and lungs.

13   Improved mood.

14   Strengthened immune system.

15   Prolonged good health and independence in seniors.

16   Better quality of life.

## How you can get started building activity into your life:

**Start slow** - The good news is, you don't have to change everything at the same time. In fact, the trick to healthy living is making small gradual changes. Take more and more steps each day, adding walking to your day, taking an extra fitness class. So, what else can you be doing to live healthy and active? Your first step on your Mission is to start moving more.

**Slowing increase intensity** - it's as easy as taking a walk around the block a few times a week. Once you get comfortable with that, walk a little further, or walk a little faster. As you progress you will want to walk at a pace as if you are late for picking up your kids or a meeting, but don't push yourself too hard. Generally, you can exercise safely if you start at an easy pace and slowly work up to a harder level. If you have not exercised for some time or want to try a harder exercise, talk to your doctor or a health care practitioner as to what exercise is best for you.

**Just get started** - We know we need to exercise, but we have so many excuses not to do it. For most people, getting started is the hardest part of regular exercise. It is recommended to have your fitness level assessed by a fitness professional, such as a personal trainer.

**Goals will help motivation** - We each have to find the motivation that works for us. Start by assessing your goals, your interests and how ready you are to begin active living. Having goals for yourself can help you stay motivated along your path. Making a commitment to lead a healthier, more active lifestyle does not mean a life of harsh discipline. It also helps to have fun.

**Pick activities that you enjoy** - The truth is, everything counts and the more you move, the healthier you'll be. See if you can discover the joy of moving. Find a dance class, if you like dancing. Find friends to golf with, if you like golfing. If you like tennis, find a friend to play tennis with. If you like hiking, get out with your dog or friend hiking.

**Find fitness buddies** - If you like, find exercise "buddies." It's always more fun and motivating to have buddies to keep you active.

**Reward your efforts** - And reward yourself for your progress. Treat yourself to a massage, a pedicure, or a leisurely library visit, a new music CD or book (that you can get inspired by).

**Simple ways to move your body** - You can increase your amount of active living. You can start the process of being healthy and losing weight now by adding a little more activity to your life. Be aware. Make a list of all the physical activities you do on a typical day. If you find that the bulk of your time is spent sitting, make another list of all the ways you could move more--getting up each hour to stretch or walk, walk the stairs at work, etc.

**Turn off the TV** - Once a week, turn off the TV and do something a little more physical with your family. Play games, take a walk... almost anything will be more active than sitting on the couch.

**Walk more** - Look for small ways to walk more. When you get the mail, take a walk around the block, take the dog for an extra outing each day or walk on your treadmill for 5 minutes before getting ready for work.

**Do some cleaning or chores** - Chores and cleaning are all ways to be more active. Chores like, shoveling snow, working in the garden, raking leaves, mopping or sweeping the floors. These kinds of activities may not be too 'vigorous', but they can keep you moving and help contribute to overall activity for your day while getting your house in order.

**Walk while you talk** - When you're on the phone, pace around or even do some cleaning while chatting. This is a great way to stay moving while doing something you enjoy. It always amazes me how long my sister or friends and I can talk. So I make maximum use of that time. Next time your friend who loves to talk calls, get your shoes on and start walking with them on the phone.

Creating a healthy lifestyle doesn't have to mean drastic changes. In fact, drastic changes almost always lead to failure. Making small changes in how you live each day can lead to big rewards, so figure out what you can do to be healthy today.

*Remember:*
*Stay true to your Mission...*

*"When diet is wrong medicine is of no use. When diet is correct medicine is of no need."*

— *Ayurveda Proverb*

# — WEEK TEN —

## Nutrition Management

Ayurveda can be your natural path to a
slim and happy life.

Ayurveda is all about finding a balance in your life. If you
are overweight, then somewhere along the line an imbalance has
occurred and weight gain is the product of the imbalance. As
mentioned numerous times, you need to take a realistic approach to
your situation; there's no magic involved - just a long hard look at
what your complete lifestyle is like and why you've become the way
you are. A reality check, if you will. According to Deepak Chopra,
the best weight loss program will improve your relationship with
your body and food. When you make choices that cause you to gain
weight, your body communicates distress signs. Through Ayurveda,

you can discover how to listen, understand and respond mindfully to these warning signs. A new relationship with food will feed your health and weight management in many ways. Weight loss is only one of the many benefits. More than a mere system of treating illness, Ayurveda is a science of life!

## What is Ayurveda?

Ayurveda medicine- also known as Ayurveda- is one of the oldest holistic or whole body system that heals. It was developed thousands of years ago and is the oldest continuously practiced health-care system. It is based on the belief that health and wellness depend on a delicate balance between your mind, body and spirit. The two main guiding principles according to Deepak Chopra, M.D., the mind and body are inextricably connected, and nothing has more power to heal and transform the body than the mind. Ayurveda is drawn from an understanding of nature's rhythms and laws. If we choose to ignore these laws, then imbalances will start to appear or show up. The primary focus of Ayurveda is to promote optimal health, instead of just fighting off disease and illness. According to Ayurveda, good health is achieved when your mind, body and spirit are in harmony or balanced. A disruption in this harmony can lead to weight gain, poor health, illness and sickness. The goal of Ayurveda is to teach people how to achieve optimal health through a deeper understanding of themselves and their own role in relationship of mind and body. It is a system based on natural healing through strengthening the body, mind and spirit and allowing the individual to activate the natural healing mechanisms to work to their fullest potential.

## What is Ayurvedic Nutrition?

It is hard to believe that something as obvious as nutrition is commonly overlooked in the modern health care system. Fortunately, there is a growing focus on the important role that nutrition can play in helping you maintain good health. In Ayurveda, food plays a prominent important role in the promotion of health and is therefore considered medicine. The Foundation of Ayurvedic Nutrition is based on the idea that you are the result of what, when, where, how and why you eat. Ayurveda explains that your food should be eaten mindfully and with gratitude, and that it must be fresh, of the highest quality, digestible, delicious, lovingly prepared and satisfying to your senses. Sounds familiar doesn't it? This reinforces many of the suggestions made already along the way on the program. Ayurveda offers a balanced approach to preparing, eating and digesting your food based on your unique body-mind type or Dosha, as well as the time of day, the season, your life-cycle and where you live. (You can discover more on your own personal Dosha, and the general qualities of how they affect your balance by researching Ayurveda deeper. Connect with The Foundation of Ayurvedic Nutrition for more on Dosha)

Ayurveda teaches us that food should be appealing, not only to your sense of taste, but also your sense of sight, smell, touch and even sound. Digestion begins with the production of enzymatic saliva in your mouth and it is all your sensory organs that stimulate this digestive process. When you use various foods and spices that are flavorful, aromatic, and appealing with an assortment of colours and textures, it makes your experience of food better and provides you with a wide range of nutrients.

Unlike a fad diet, the dietary practices in Ayurveda encourage a conscious way of living and eating. Ayurveda is a way of embracing food as life-giving fuel. Ayurveda explains that your dietary needs and your digestion are affected by nature and the changes that occur in your life. It is a holistic approach to life and eating. Living an Ayurvedic lifestyle is to make food choices that are based on the quality of the food, the current season and your location. It is all about the what, when and how we eat that is important. Ayurveda encourages you to prepare and eat your food in a peaceful, loving and positive environment. Also, it is important to greet your food with reverence and acknowledge its source with gratitude.

### How you can lose weight with Ayurveda?

If you're serious about losing weight, Ayurveda, provides balancing health benefits, that can bring impressive results and often that means regulating your metabolism. While adopting Ayurveda practices is about much more than losing weight, there are some quick fix Ayurveda alterations you can make to your lifestyle that can help you with sustained weight-loss. Although different people have weight issues for different reasons these what, when and how tips, could help. Losing weight naturally encompasses bringing a balanced change into your diet, exercise and lifestyle patterns. What, when and how you eat is the key to losing weight with Ayurveda nutrition.

What to eat- In Ayurveda it is suggested that the best medicine is food harvested in-season. Some animals naturally eat a high protein, high fat diet in the winter, emphasizing nuts and grains. Nature provides us humans a similar suggestion to the cold of winter with soups, stews, meats, grains and fats. It is the high protein, high fat time of year. In the spring, the season changes. It is a rainy, cool season. Nature again provides the antidote with low fat, mucous reducing foods such as leafy greens, sprouts, berries, root veggies and grapefruits. All these foods are fat-burning and detoxification and cleansing foods, making them perfect for spring. In the summer, the rules change once again. During the hot summer months, nature brings with it cool fruits and veggies to help keep us from getting too hot and dried out. Try not to think of what not to eat but rather think of what to eat more of. Certain foods are better for you when they are in season. Having a wide variety of food is good for nutrition and to prevent the body from developing food cravings. Food cravings often occur because of imbalanced diets.

Drink hot water frequently throughout the day- By sipping hot water throughout the day you help cleanse the digestive tract and entire body of blockages and impurities. Hot water drinking improves digestion and assimilation of food and helps prevent the body from becoming toxic and clogged. It also is a great aid in reducing food cravings between meals. I have known people who lost over 50 pounds by following only this single recommendation. I usually recommend getting a thermos and bring it with you, sip it during the day. You can pour your hot water in the cup and sip it throughout the day as you work.

When to eat- According to Ayurvedic Nutrition, to begin the weight loss process, try eating three substantial meals a day without between-meal snacks. This will begin to nudge your blood sugar's ability to make energy last from one meal to the next. It is the Ayurveda philosophy that in between meals, your body burns fat, which is your stable, non-emergency fuel. If you snack then, there is no need for your body to burn its stored fat. If you are stressed, your body sends the signal to store fat and crave sugar, which is not good for managing weight and balancing your body. Eat a light evening meal with easy-to-digest foods. If you continue to eat large evening meals with heavy foods it is virtually impossible to make serious progress according to Ayurveda nutrition. I cannot emphasize this point too much. Ayurveda describes that digestion is less strong in the evening, plus lying down to sleep a few hours later further slows down digestion, metabolism and circulation. This reinforces the suggestions made in week two on your Mission! The body simply cannot assimilate large evening meals properly. The result is that most of the food is digested poorly and eventually creates toxins, fat and excess weight. According to Ayurveda Nutrition, evening meals should be light or vegetarian, hot, light and liquid like if possible. As your blood sugars start to become more stable, you will notice how your hunger level in the evening becomes less strong. Slowly, as it becomes easier, begin to eat an earlier and lighter dinner. It is through this process that you will give your body permission to burn fat instead of sugar and carbs. Eat the largest meal of the day at lunch if possible to promote fat burning at night and regulate blood sugar levels during the day. Lunch is the time our bodies can digest and assimilate well due to the fact that digestion is strongest at noon and we have many active hours to metabolize the food before we sleep. Lunch is the most important meal of the day according to Ayurvedic Nutrition. Lunch should be warm, cooked foods with a wide variety of tastes and dishes. Warm food is essential as it can be more easily digested and assimilated. Cold foods suppress digestion. A good, balanced lunch also helps us feel less hungry in the evening, making it easier to stick to that important light evening meal.

How to eat- Sitting down and eating a meal is becoming more and more rare these days. When I traveled to Europe, I noticed they often sit down for every meal. They rarely had to go cups for my morning tea. They relax, dine and enjoy well prepared food in a relaxed social setting. In our North American society we tend to eat in our cars on the way to gymnastics or in front of the TV. This disconnect between mind and body while eating is harmful. When you are relaxed, the digestive process is more effective. It is important according to Ayurvedic nutrition, that you are relaxed when eating, then the mind and body become nourished, and you can experience the taste of the food and assimilate the mental, physical and spiritual benefits of a balanced meal.

Health is won or lost in how we live day-to-day life. Today take the initiative and get on an upward spiral closer and closer to healthy living.

## Ayurveda tips for balanced living:

(According to New England Institute of Ayurvedic Medicine)
Beneficial Daily Routines

1. Rise before the sunrise.
2. Drink a full glass (8 oz.) of room temperature or warm water.
3. Clean your face, mouth and nasal passages and gargle with salt water.
4. Do some light yoga or stretching exercises.
5. Meditate for 20 minutes.
6. Take a walk or run for ½ hour, 3–4 times per week.
7. Have a nutritional breakfast according to your body type.
8. Have a relaxing or complete meal at lunchtime. 11–2 pm.
9. Relax for ½ hour after lunch.
10. Meditate in late afternoon before evening meal for 20 minutes.
11. Eat dinner between 5:00 and 7:00 pm. This should not be a heavy meal.
12. Allow two hours after your dinner before going to bed.
13. Bedtime 10:00–11:00 pm.
14. Give thanks.

You have many nutritional and lifestyle tools that can all work synergistically to help you attain your weight loss and weight management goals. What worked well for you on the program? Make those adjustments a permanent part of your lifestyle. You are special, and you will leave a legacy behind you. Be the person you want to be and make a positive impression in this world. Focus on what you do well, the positive trail you leave, and what makes you special and unique. Since this program is based on naturally balancing your weight, many of the protocols have now become a part of your life naturally. Your effort along your Mission has paid off and continues to benefit you on a deep level. Start to acknowledge you are not that bad and you deserve to be loved. Begin to love, nurture, and care for yourself on a regular basis. Listen to your dreams and requests. Respect your own wishes and wants. Praise yourself for just being you! Live in confidence and happiness, don't sell yourself short, you deserve the best for yourself.

# STAY
# ON TARGET

## MY WEEKLY CHECKLIST

- ☑ Praise yourself
- ☑ Stay on your Mission
- ☑ Make a list of what worked
- ☑ Create positive self talk
- ☐ _____
- ☐ _____
- ☐ _____
- ☐ _____
- ☐ _____
- ☐ _____
- ☐ _____
- ☐ _____
- ☐ _____
- ☐ _____
- ☐ _____
- ☐ _____
- ☐ _____

## MY WEIGHT THIS WEEK:

Began at:_____

Finished at:_____

Total weight loss:_____

## MY MEASUREMENTS THIS WEEK:

### BEGAN AT

Shoulders:_____

Chest:_____

Waist:_____

Hips:_____

### FINISHED AT

Shoulders:_____

Chest:_____

Waist:_____

Hips:_____

### DIFFERENCE/TOTAL INCHES LOST:

Shoulders:_____

Chest:_____

Waist:_____

Hips:_____

What really resonated for me this week?

_____
_____
_____
_____
_____
_____
_____
_____
_____
_____

What worked well for me this week?

_____
_____
_____
_____
_____
_____
_____
_____
_____
_____
_____

"*Do not go where the path may lead,
go instead where there is no path and
leave a trail*"

— *Ralph Waldo Emerson*

## Mission Slim Possible Summary:

- Natural, nutrient dense foods are the secret to shedding weight and keeping your weight and health managed properly.
- The two most highly processed products that are consumed are sugar and wheat.
- Natural sweeteners are foods with nutritional value and natural fiber.
- Wheat products are mass produced and mass consumed. Grains, such as wheat, are spoiled if they are not in their natural state.
- The eating of grains in their natural state - the state that nature intended - has a positive, profound effect on health and weight management. Whole grains are full of nutritional value and enter your body with full fiber and nutrients.
- You create your own reality with your thoughts, feelings and attitudes.
- When you consume alive foods you can't help but feel full of life. Alive foods also contain a large amount of nutrients with low calories.
- Good quality foods will change the quality of your life.
- A day of cleansing to saturate your body with nutrition is a good tool to use to improve health on all levels and manage weight.
- You can use the power of affirmations to create everything you desire for yourself.
- By slowing down and eating mindfully, you not only improve digestion but you eat fewer calories.
- Smart sizing (portion control) is a natural way to permanently decrease your calories and still consume the things you like.
- The power of visualization is an effective tool that is as easy as daydreaming. By creating a picture of your goals in your mind

and keeping that image fixed in your mental construct, you have the capability to turn that image into a reality.

- Diet now and you will gain weight later.
- We need good quality fat in our diet for many health reasons and also weight management.
- We need fat for many health reasons and also for weight management.
- Boost your metabolism by eating more frequently, sleep well, drink water, exercise, increase muscle mass on your body and eat from all food categories. Sea vegetables boost thyroid function too.
- Jump into life with both feet, take action and get the results you are looking for.
- Controlling stress and cortisol levels is clearly critical to achieving our overall goals of shedding extra body weight.
- Being optimistic can lead you to feel better about yourself and the accomplishments you have made.
- There are advantages to planning your meals ahead. Follow your plans and you can achieve your goals.
- Move it and you will lose it: walk the pounds away and stay healthy.
- You need to honor and celebrate the achievements you have made and the successful strides you have achieved.
- The secret to losing weight and staying slim and healthy is to gain control of your life. Now is the time to direct your food choices and feel empowered as a result. Eliminate your trigger foods.
- Slim and Healthy is not free; it requires your efforts.
- Blood sugar levels can greatly affect our weight management efforts. By choosing natural, nutrient dense fiber rich foods

that are low on the glycemic index, you can regulate mood, energy and weight.

- Notice your small successes and let compliments others give you flow into your bones.
- Choose the natural path to manage your weight with Ayurveda.
- Each day keep a log of what you are grateful for about YOU.

### Where to go from here:

Invest in yourself & your dreams. You can have the life you desire. Is it time to finally make those changes that you've been dreaming of? Would you like to break free from procrastination, and finally keep those promises to yourself? Would you like to bring your life into wonderful, purposeful, healthy balance? Would you like to take your dreams in your heart, and finally take the steps to bring them into reality? Make your self and your life a priority, it's time! Moving forward take all the tools from Mission Slim Possible that have worked well for you and bring them into the future. If you follow your most courageous, authentic path, you'll usually end up astounding and impressing everyone around you, no matter how much they didn't understand, or tried to discourage you, at the beginning. Follow your desires, goals and purpose and you will be pleased with your progress. Go There! Mission Slim Possible: 10 Week Diet Revenge has helped you find your unique path to personal success with an action-oriented emphasis on accountability, resourcefulness and wellness. Your game plan for the future is up to you. Create what matters most in your life. Wake up your inner warrior and keep your focus on your desires and goals and you will continue to be successful on all levels.

**Find your inner hero and continue to follow its courage:**

*"Inner Hero Pledge" Annonymous*

- To do what's right . . . even if you are afraid.
- To listen to the inner wisdom . . . and not the random opinions of others.
- To be kind . . . and remember that sometimes the person you need to be the kindest to is yourself.
- To live by choice . . . not chance.
- To pursue excellence . . . excel, but not compete.
- To have integrity . . . keep your word and your commitments to others.
- To make corrections and changes . . . not make excuses.
- To be fair and treat all people with respect, and understand their point of view. . . even if you don't agree with it.

"Most of all being a hero means accepting yourself with a deep kindness that makes a positive difference in your life. Live your authentic life and keep making targets for yourself. By moving forward with optimism, courage and heroism you will allow for a future of good health, happiness and success on all levels. Wishing you strength, courage and success."

- Andrea Seydel

**Andrea Seydel** is a Nutritionist (RD) and Certified Life Coach (ICF), Can-Fit-Pro, LesMills, Pilates, Yoga and Zumba certified fitness instructor. She received her B.A. in Psychology from York University and concluded post-graduate work in Positive Psychology. Andrea is the founder of Life Balance Publishing Group, where she publishes various magazines, books and newsletters all relating to balancing and improving lives. Andrea's passion to help others recognize and tap into their potential to live their best life is seen in her writing, classes, and presentations. Her enthusiasm and passion, combined with her health and fitness knowledge make self improvement almost contagious. When Andrea is not on one of her own personal mission's, she loves to spend her time hiking the trails with her rescue dog, doing yoga and being with her two kids in Caledon, Ontario.

*"Helping you get diet revenge"*

— *Andrea Seydel*

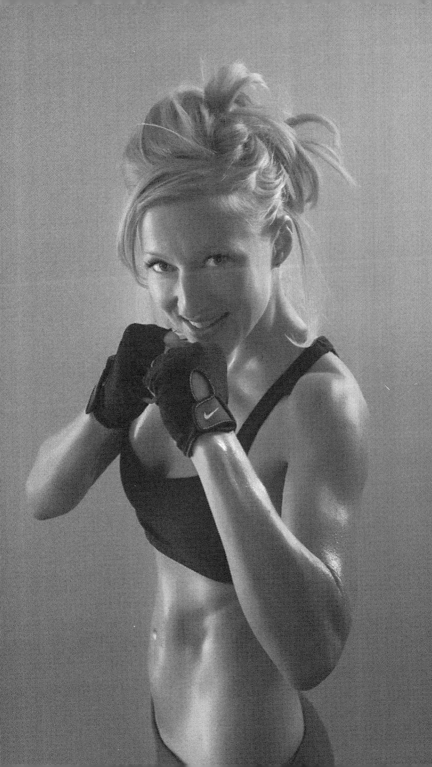

# ON LINE WORKS CONSULTED AND CITED

http://www.grainchain.com/Resources/11-14/ip_wheat-into-flour-the-milling-process ("650 million tons of wheat is produced around the world. It is one of the most important products feeding our world today")

http://www.hc-sc.gc.ca/fn-an/nutrition/whole-grain-entiers-eng.php

http://thespeltbakers.ca/what-is-spelt/: The benefits of spelt

http://www.ontariohoney.ca/

http://www.myfitnesspal.com/food/calories/brosia-canada-raw-honey-1539666

http://abcnews.go.com/Health/Diet/arsenic-organics-rice/story?id=15642428

http://www.soilandhealth.org/01aglibrary/010120albrecht.usdayrbk/lsom.html (Soil article)

http://www.webmd.com/diet/high-protein-low-carbohydrate-diets?page=2

http://kidshealth.org/teen/your_body/body_basics/metabolism.html#

Author, Ken Blanchard in What Your Doctor May Not Tell You About Hypothyroidism,

http://en.wikipedia.org/wiki/Whole_grain

https://www.cocomamafoods.com/ingredient-glossary/

Experience magazine - Fall 2013

http://stress.about.com/od/stresshealth/a/cortisol.htm

http://faculty.clintoncc.suny.edu/faculty/michael.gregory/files/bio%20
102/bio%20102%20lectures/digestive%20system/digestive%20system.
htm (Digestion)

Eating Free: The Carb-Friendly Way to Lose Inches, Embrace Your
Hunger, and Keep Weight Off for Good

http://www.hitchedmag.com/print.php?id=1108

http://nyxstium.info/tag/abuse/

http://www.positivityblog.com/index.php/2009/10/09/how-to-break-
out-of-a-victim-mentality-7-powerful-tips/

http://www.betterhealth.vic.gov.au/bhcv2/bhcarticles.nsf/pages/
Physical_activity_tips_to_overcome_the_barriers?open

http://life.gaiam.com/article/12-tips-fit-exercise-your-day

http://www.mayoclinic.org/fitness/art-20044531

http://www.huguenard.net/the_benefits_of_family_meal_
planning_192722a.html

http://www.extension.iastate.edu/foodsavings/page/prepare-food-ahead

http://www.psychologicalselfhelp.org

http://www.artofmanliness.com/2010/09/07/never-let-the-sun-catch-
you-sleeping-why-and-how-to-become-an-early-riser/

http://www.discovergoodnutrition.com/2012/11/early-morning-workout/

http://www.nutritionist-resource.org.uk/articles/controlling-cravings.html

http://getyouinshape.wordpress.com/category/weight-loss/page/36/

http://www.hughston.com/hha/a_15_2_5.htm

chopra.com/ccl/what-is-ayurveda

www.bodybuilding.com.

www.freeaffirmations.org

http://www.webmd.com/diet/features/lose-weight-while-sleeping?page=1

http://www.canfitpro.com

http://www.goodlifefitness.com

# WORKS CITED

Ainsworth, B.E., Haskell, W.L., Leon, A.S. Jacobs, D.R., Montoye, H.J., Sallis, J.F. & Parffenbarger, R.S. (1993). Compendium of Physical activities: Classification of energy costs of human physical activities. Medicine and Science in Sports and Exercise, 25, 71-80.

Ajzen, I., & Fishbein, M. (1980). Understanding attitudes and predicting social behavior. Englewood Cliffs, NJ: Prentice-Hall.

Allison, D. B., & Faith, M. S. (1996). Hypnosis as an adjunct to cognitive-behavioral psychotherapy for obesity: A meta-analytic reappraisal. Journal of Consulting and Clinical Psychology, 64, 513 -516.

American Medical Association, (1993). Very low-calorie diets. Journal of the American Medical Association, 270, 967-974.

Axe, Dr. Josh, The Health Virus Jan 1, 2009.

Bandura, A. (1977). Self-efficacy: Toward a unifying theory of behavioral change. Psychological Review, 84, 191-215.

Bandura, A. (1991c). Social cognitive theory of self-regulation. Organizational Behavior and Human Decision Processes, 50, 248-287.

Brown, A. L. (1984). Metacognition, executive control, self-regulation, and other even more mysterious mechanisms. In F. E. Weinert & R. H. Kluwe (Eds.), Metacognition, motivation, and learning (pp. 60-108). Stuttgart, West Germany: Kuhlhammer.

Brownell, K.D., & Wadden, T.A. (1992). Etiology and treatment of obesity: understanding a serious, prevalent, and refractory disorder. Special Issue: Behavioral medicine: An update for the 1990's. Journal of Consulting and Clinical Psychology, 60, 505-517.

Brownell, K. D., & Stunkard, A. J. (1980). Physical activity in the development and control of obesity. In A. J. Stunkard (Ed.), Obesity (pp. 300-324). Philadelphia, PA: W. B. Saunders Co.

Bulik, C.M. (1992). Abuse of drugs associated with eating disorders. Journal of Substance Abuse, 4, 6990.

Calder, B. J., & Staw, B. M. (1975). Self-perception of intrinsic and extrinsic motivation. Journal of Personality and Social Psychology, 31, 599-605.

Carroll, W. R., & Bandura, A. (1987). Translating cognition into action: The role of visual guidance in observational learning. Journal of Motor Behavior, 19, 385-398.

Centers for Disease Control (1996). Adverse Events Associated with EphedrineContaining Products  Texas, December 1993September 1995.

DiCicco, Tony., Catch Them Being Good: Everything You Need to Know to Successfully Coach Girls. Viking USA. Aug., 2002.

Morbidity and Mortality Weekly Report, 45, 689693.

Champlin, T. S. (1977). Self-deception: A reflexive dilemma. Philosophy, 52, 281-299.

Dollard, J., & Miller, N. E. (1950). Personality and psychotherapy. New York: McGraw-Hill.

Duda (1988). The relationship between goal perspectives, persistence and behavioral intensity among male and female recreational sport participants. Leisure Sciences, 10, 95-106.

Earley, P. C., Connolly, T., & Lee, C. (1989). Task strategy interventions in goal setting: The importance of search in strategy development. Journal of Management, 15, 589-602.

Dyer, W., Wayne, Wishes Fulfilled, Hay House April 4, 2012.

Evans, David Patchell., Living the Good Life: Your Guide to Health and Success, ECW Press, 2004.

George, T. R., Feltz, D. L., & Chase, M. A. (1992). Effects of model similarity on self-efficacy and muscular endurance: A second-look. Journal of Sport & Exercise Psychology, 14, 237-248.

Hagan, Maureen, Newbody Workout For Women- 6 Weeks to a Fit and Fabulous New You. Dec 29, 2009. Penguin Canada.

Hall, H. K., & Byrne, A. T. J. (1988). Goal setting in sport: Clarifying recent anomalies. Journal of Sport & Exercise Psychology, 10, 184-198.

Hans, Selye., Stress of Life Magraw-Hill Inc. 1978.

Hay, Louise, You Can Heal Your Life Hay House, Jan 1, 1984.

Hay, Louise, and Richardson, Cheryl, You can Create An Exceptional Life Hay House, Jan 8, 2013.

Heska, S., Feld, K., & Yang, M.U. (1993). Resting energy expenditure in the obese: A cross-validation and comparison of prediction equations. Journal of the American Dietetic Association, 93, 1031-1036.

Kinney, J.M. (1995). Influence of altered body weight on energy expenditure. Nutrition Reviews, 53, 265-268.

Kirsch, 1. (1996). Hypnotic enhancement of cognitive-behavioral weight loss treatmentsAnother meta-reanalysis. Jourml of Consulting @ Clinical Psychology, 64, 517-519.

Krantz, S. E. (1985). When depressive cognitions reflect negative realities. Cognitive Therapy and Research, 9, 595-610.

Kuczmarski RJ, Flegal KM, Campbell SM, Johnson CL. Increasing prevalence of overweight among U.S. adults: the National Health and Nutrition Examination Surveys, 19601991. JAMA 1994;272:20511.

Langer, E. J. (1983). The psychology of control. California: Sage Publications.

Little, B. L., & Madigan, R. M. (1994, August). Motivation in work teams: A test of the construct of collective efficacy. Paper presented at the annual meeting of the Academy of Management, Houston, TX.

Margolis, D. (1995). Weight loss products. American health, 14, 14-15.

Mathews, A., & Milroy, R. (1994). Effects of priming and suppression of worry. Behaviour Research and Therapy, 32, 843-850.

Miller, S. M. (1980). Why having control reduces stress: If I can stop the rollercoaster I don't want to get off. In J. Garber & M. E. P. Seligman (Eds.), Human helplessness: Theory and applications (pp. 71-95). New York: Academic Press.

Morgan, J.P., Funderburk, F.R., Blackburn, G.L., Noble, R. (1989). Subjective profile of phenylpropanolamine: Absence of stimulant or euphorigenic effects at recommended dose levels. Journal of Clinical Psychopharmacology, 9, 3338.

Nicholls, J. G. (1984). Achievement motivation: Conceptions of ability, subjective experience, task choice, and performance. Psychological Review, 91, 328-346.

Phares, E. J. (1976). Locus of control in personality. Morristown, NJ: General Learning Press.

Powers, W. T. (1973). Behavior: The control of perception. Chicago: Aldine.

Rogers, R. W. (1983). Cognitive and physiological processes in fear appeals and attitude change: A revised theory of protection motivation. In J. T. Cacioppo & R. E. Petty (Eds.), Social psychophysiology (pp. 153-176). New York: Guildford Press.

Rosenberg, Marshall. Nonviolent Communication- A language Of Life. Puddle Dancer, 2003.

Ryan, T. A. (1970). Intentional behavior. New York: Ronald Press.

Rubin, R. (1994). The cost of weight loss. American health, 13, 91.

Shapiro, Debbie, Your Body Speaks Your Mind: Decoding the Emotional, Psychological, and Spiritual Messages That Underlie Illness Sounds True Incorporated, April 1, 2005.

Siegel, Dr. Bernie, A Book of Miracles New World Library, Sept. 20, 2011.

Shovic, A.C., Adams, A.S., & Dubitzky, J. (1993). Effectiveness and dropout rate of a very-low calorie diet program. Journal of the American Dietetic Association, 93, 583-584.

Swami, Satchidananda. The Yoga Sutras of Patanjali, Schocken Books. 1976.

Thompson, J., & Manore, M.M. (1996). Predicted and measured resting metabolic rate of male and female endurance athletes. Journal of the American Dietetic Association, 96, 30-34.

U.S. Department of Health and Human Services (1988). Healthy people 2000: National health promotion and disease prevention objectives. Washington: Public Health Service.

Vanherweghem, J.L., Depierreux, M., & Christian, T. (1993). Rapidly progressing interstitial renal fibrosis in young women: Association with slimming regimen including Chinese Herbs. Lancet, 341, 387-391.

Wellman, P.J., & Sellers, T.L. (1986). Weight loss induced by chronic phenylpropanolamine: Anorexia and brown adipose tissue thermogenesis. Pharmacology, Biochemistry and Behavior, 24,605611.

For Mission Slim Possible: 10 Week Diet
Revenge online support and guidance visit

www.andreaseydel.com

Made in the USA
Charleston, SC
21 November 2014